THE ART OF NURSING

A CELEBRATION OF OUR PROFESSION

Baptist Health South Florida

Curated by Yvonne Brookes, R.N. • Photography by Fareed Al-Mashat • Edited by Timothy Dodson

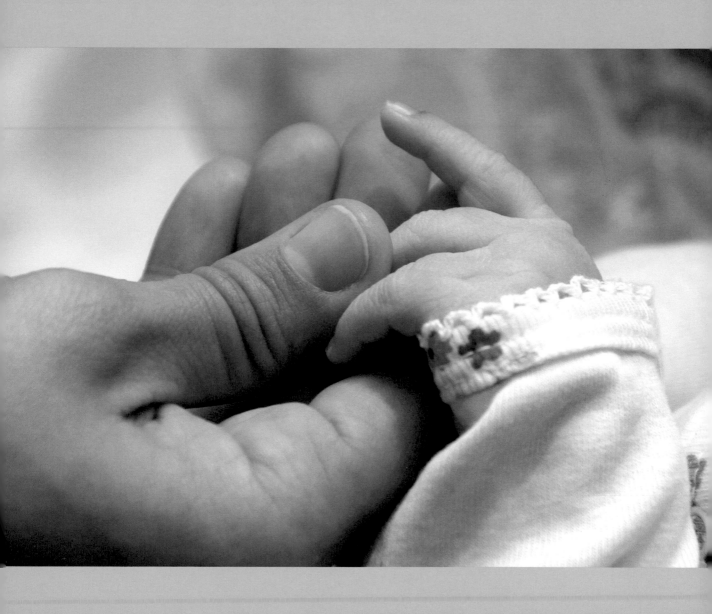

Anyone can be trained to bandage a leg, give medication or handle an IV; the true calling of a nurse is to help heal the whole person. Nurses display a unique set of qualities that position them to connect with another human who not only needs help with a physical condition, but also needs someone to touch his heart.

YVONNE BROOKES, R.N.

Copyright © 2013
Baptist Health South Florida

Published by
Baptist Health South Florida

Printed in the United States

Library of Congress
Control Number
2013931880

Baptist Health South Florida:
The Art of Nursing
1. Medicine – Nursing – Florida
ISBN 978-1-4675-6392-5

CURATOR
Yvonne Brookes, R.N.

PHOTOGRAPHER
Fareed Al-Mashat

EDITOR
Timothy Dodson

GRAPHIC DESIGN
Rhondda Edmiston
Mixed Media, Inc.

PHOTOGRAPHY-DESIGN
Alla Katsenovich

PRODUCTION ASSISTANT
Andra Ogden Demorizi

BAPTIST HEALTH SOUTH FLORIDA
MARKETING & PUBLIC RELATIONS

Roymi V. Membiela
Corporate Vice President

Georgina Gonzalez-Robiou, APR
Director

Address inquiries to:
Baptist Health South Florida
6855 Red Road
Coral Gables, FL 33143
TheArtofNursing@BaptistHealth.net

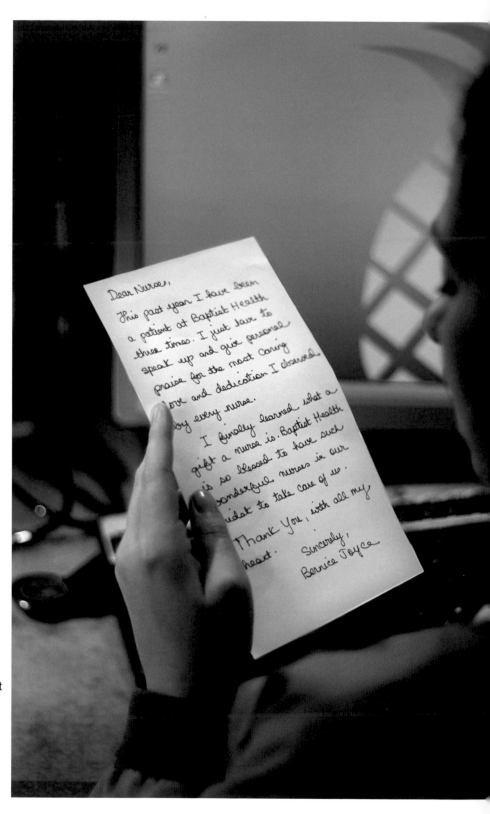

TABLE OF CONTENTS

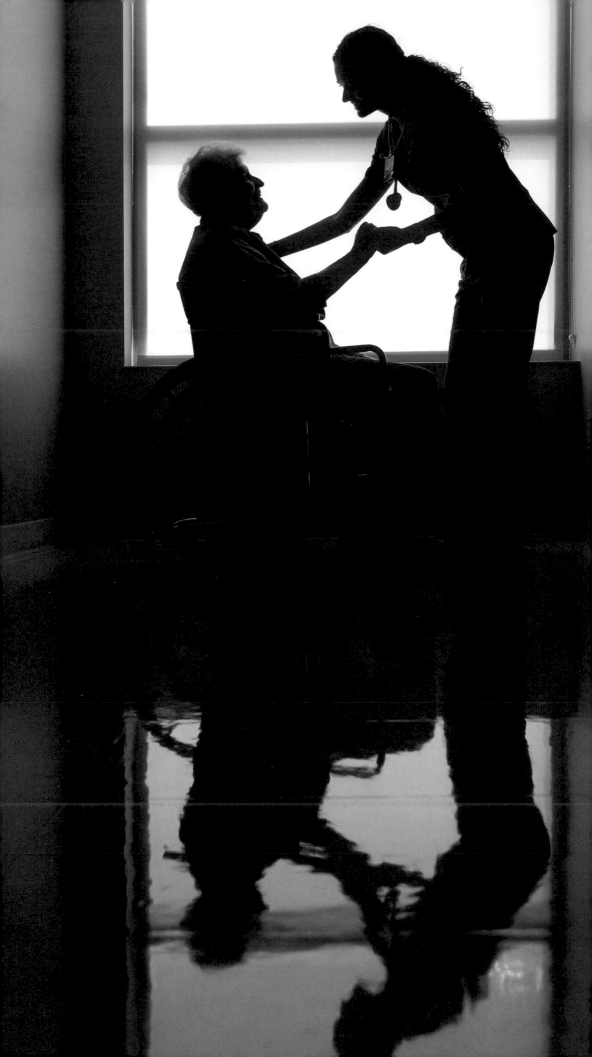

urses have always been the heart of Baptist Health South Florida. Since the formation of Baptist Health in 1990 — indeed, since the founding of some of our original facilities in the 1940s — nurses have answered their calling to reach out to those in need and care for our community. Every day, in countless ways, Baptist Health nurses help to fulfill our mission: to improve the health and well-being of individuals, and to promote the sanctity and preservation of life, in the communities we serve.

The practice of nursing has undergone many changes in recent years, both within our organization and across the nation. Today's nurses not only have met these challenges, they also have discovered a wealth of opportunities to have an even greater impact on the delivery of healthcare across the continuum of life. They have risen to the highest levels of leadership within healthcare organizations, bringing along the next generation of caregivers. Scientific and technological advances have opened doors for nurses to focus on exciting specialties or pursue careers as educators or researchers. Yet, it is not the science, but the art of nursing that we explore in this book.

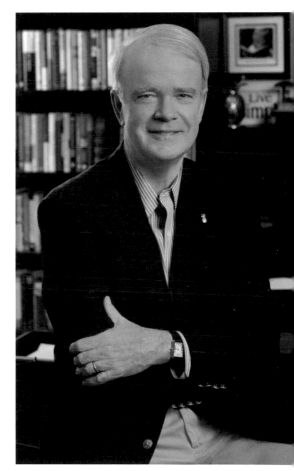

Nurses understand instinctively that patients and their families must be our partners in the healing process. Baptist Health's focus on patient- and family-centered care highlights the nurse's role as listener, critical thinker, collaborator and advocate.

On behalf of Baptist Health South Florida, I salute our nurses for the skill and compassion with which they practice their art.

Brian E. Keeley
President and Chief Executive Officer
Baptist Health South Florida

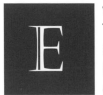

Every nurse's story is different, yet every story is the same. Throughout my career as a nurse, and particularly during my time with Baptist Health South Florida, I have heard hundreds of stories of women and men who have been drawn to this profession of caring and compassion.

Some discover their calling to care for others as small children, taking a temperature or bandaging the injuries of a wounded doll. Others come to nursing much later in life, often after years in a successful career in an entirely unrelated field.

Many are fortunate to have gained firsthand knowledge of nursing because of a friend or relative who worked in healthcare. Others, sadly, became caregivers themselves during the illness or death of a beloved family member.

Regardless of the personal path that leads to the profession, there is a certain set of core attributes and values present in almost all nurses. *The Art of Nursing*, based on a 2011 Baptist Health photo exhibition of the same name, explores these common traits through compelling images and the words of our own Baptist Health nurses. Yvonne Brookes, Baptist Health's director of clinical learning, and Fareed Al-Mashat, one of our most seasoned photographers, were inspired to create these photographs to capture the rich diversity of our nursing staff.

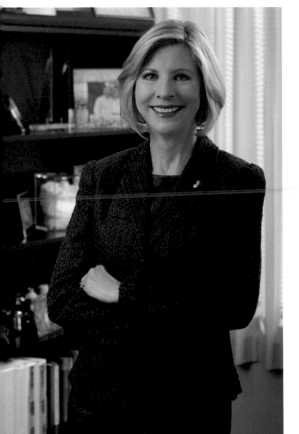

If you are a nurse, I am sure you will identify instantly with the thoughts shared in these pages. If you are contemplating a career in nursing, you will find much to inspire and motivate you. If you are not a nurse, you will gain insight into what makes us tick, and why surveys consistently name our profession the most trusted in the country.

Deborah Mulvihill

Deborah Mulvihill, R.N.
Chief Nursing Officer and Corporate Vice President
Baptist Health South Florida

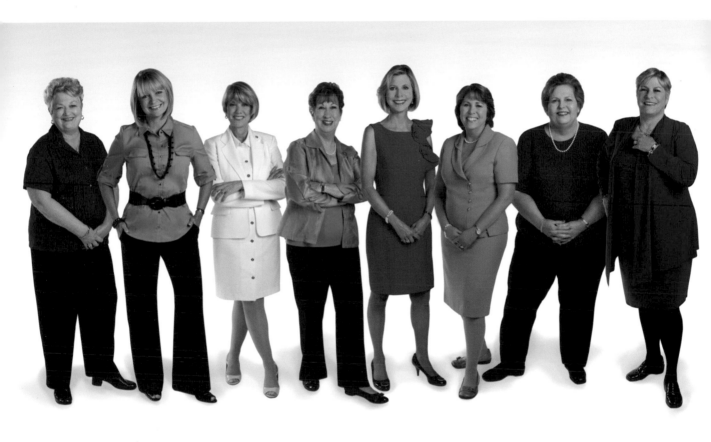

Baptist Health Chief Nursing Officers

Left to right:
Sandy Hyatt, R.N., Doctors Hospital
Tina Jones, R.N., Baptist Outpatient Services
Denise Harris, R.N., West Kendall Baptist Hospital
Kathy Sparger, R.N., South Miami Hospital
Deborah Mulvihill, R.N., Baptist Health South Florida
Cheryl Cottrell, R.N., Mariners Hospital
Gail Gordon, R.N., Homestead Hospital
Becky Montesino, R.N., Baptist Hospital of Miami

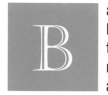aptist Health South Florida was officially created in 1990 by bringing a dynamic offering of leading-edge medical care to the community. For the first time, the region's top not-for-profit hospitals were housed under one name, with a shared mission: "to improve the health and well-being of individuals, and promote the sanctity and preservation of life."

The Baptist Health tradition of medical quality actually dates back to the 1940s, when some of its South Florida member hospitals were founded. Today, the Baptist Health network of services extends throughout Miami-Dade, Monroe and Broward counties and beyond. More than 12,000 people from 85 countries now travel to South Florida each year to receive world-class treatment from the Baptist team.

Baptist Health has built a culture of quality that extends throughout the organization. There is an overriding commitment to best-in-class customer service and an expectation of ethical performance at every level, in each location. Patient safety goes hand in hand with this culture of quality, and Baptist Health has earned the community's trust and respect.

Team members in all areas work toward a shared vision: "Baptist Health will be the preeminent healthcare provider in the communities we serve, the organization that people instinctively turn to for their healthcare needs. Baptist Health will offer a broad range of clinical services that are evidence-based and compassionately provided to ensure patient safety, superior clinical outcomes and the highest levels of satisfaction. Baptist Health will be a national and international leader in healthcare innovation."

Baptist Health is the largest faith-based, not-for-profit healthcare organization in the region. Its network comprises Baptist Hospital, South Miami Hospital, Baptist Children's Hospital, Baptist Cardiac & Vascular Institute, Homestead Hospital, Mariners Hospital, Doctors Hospital, West Kendall Baptist Hospital and Baptist Outpatient Services. Baptist Health Foundation, the organization's fundraising arm, supports services at all hospitals and facilities affiliated with Baptist Health. For more information or to explore career opportunities, visit BaptistHealth.net.

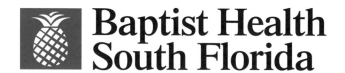

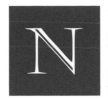 urses' decisions save lives. Their words enlighten. Their compassion eases pain. And their cheers celebrate success. They are the dedicated nurses of Baptist Health, and they provide high-quality care to patients in hospitals, outpatient facilities and even in patients' homes.

Patients and their families say "thank you" to nurses every day, and the Baptist Health staff feels appreciated when they are acknowledged for a job well done. There are times, though, when one would like to do more than say thanks — and a donation to the **Center for Excellence in Nursing** shows the nurses who have been so important that their efforts have not gone unnoticed.

Donations to the Center are used for education and development of the nursing staff, to recognize outstanding nurses for their contributions to the profession, to send students through nursing school and to improve patient care with nurse-approved equipment and programs.

Proceeds from the sale of this book benefit the Baptist Health South Florida **Center for Excellence in Nursing**. To learn more or make a donation, visit BaptistHealth.net/Foundation.

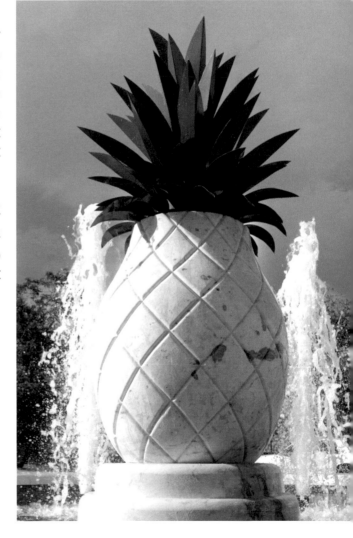

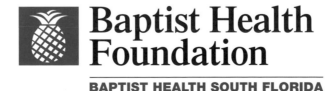

Baptist Health
Foundation

BAPTIST HEALTH SOUTH FLORIDA

CURATOR'S STATEMENT

The idea for *The Art of Nursing* grew out of a most unlikely source: a slide presentation I assembled to accompany my lecture at a nursing conference in 2010 to promote Baptist Health's South Florida RN Residency program. I searched unsuccessfully for images that conveyed the diversity and enthusiasm exhibited by the residency program's participants. So, I turned to Baptist Health photographer and video producer Fareed Al-Mashat for help.

Fareed brought some of our nurse residents into his studio for our first photo shoot, and the results exceeded my expectations. I began to think about the power of photography to express the core values of nurses and the attributes that define our profession.

In my travels around Baptist Health's various facilities, I began to collect ideas by asking nurses and patients, "give me one word that says 'nursing' to you." Their thoughtful responses led to a photo exhibition, titled *The Art of Nursing*, presented at South Miami Hospital, Baptist Hospital and West Kendall Baptist Hospital in 2011 and at Mariners Hospital in 2012.

The exhibitions struck a chord with audiences because they depict real Baptist Health nurses in realistic situations. I am so pleased that we were able to create this book to preserve the photographs for future generations of nurses to enjoy.

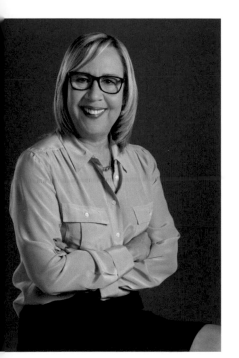

I would like to thank all the nurses of Baptist Health and, indeed, all the nurses of the world. The images in this book are my way of honoring our work, and they express my gratitude for being part of such a noble profession.

Yvonne Brookes
Yvonne Brookes, R.N.

PHOTOGRAPHER'S STATEMENT

Capturing the lives of nurses in imagery is no easy task. Because of the limitations of shooting in a hospital setting, patient privacy issues and the ever-changing daily challenges facing nurses, using a true photojournalistic approach was often not feasible. Instead, I drew on my experience as a filmmaker to capture the images by applying a controlled and staged approach to shooting, not unlike the production techniques and methods used in producing a dramatic film.

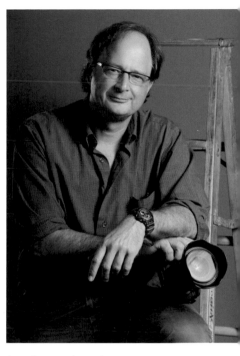

I imagined many of these images as a split second in a film sequence, then considered how I would stage, light, frame and direct that moment in time. Many of the shots were developed through a detailed storyboarding process. We strived to make these images feel as authentic and believable as if they were shot by a photojournalist.

The nurses depicted in these photos are all working professionals employed by Baptist Health South Florida. I am grateful for the personal time they devoted to our often intense photo shoots, as well as for the medical and technical expertise they offered to ensure that every photo depicted their daily reality.

Many of these images would never have come to fruition without the support of graphic designer Alla Katsenovich. Alla's creativity, precision and attention to detail helped me fully execute my photographic vision. I also thank Andra Ogden Demorizi for her assistance with logistics and schedule coordination.

Finally, I thank Yvonne Brookes, whose love for her chosen profession was the genesis of this book. A collaborator in the best sense of the word, Yvonne challenged me with her concepts and allowed me complete creative freedom to execute them.

Fareed Al-Mashat

"NURSING IS AN ART,

and if it is to be made an art, it requires an exclusive devotion, as hard a preparation, as any painter's or sculptor's work; for what is the having to do with dead canvas or dead marble, compared with having to do with the living body, the temple of God's spirit? It is one of the Fine Arts: I had almost said the finest of Fine Arts. **"**

Florence Nightingale

possessing great physical, moral or intellectual power...

STRONG

"Leaders must not only convince others to follow willingly, they must engage their team members to a degree that enables them to take charge and grow into leaders themselves. Great leaders, in a way, make their own job extinct."

SANDRA MCLEAN, R.N.

LEADERSHIP

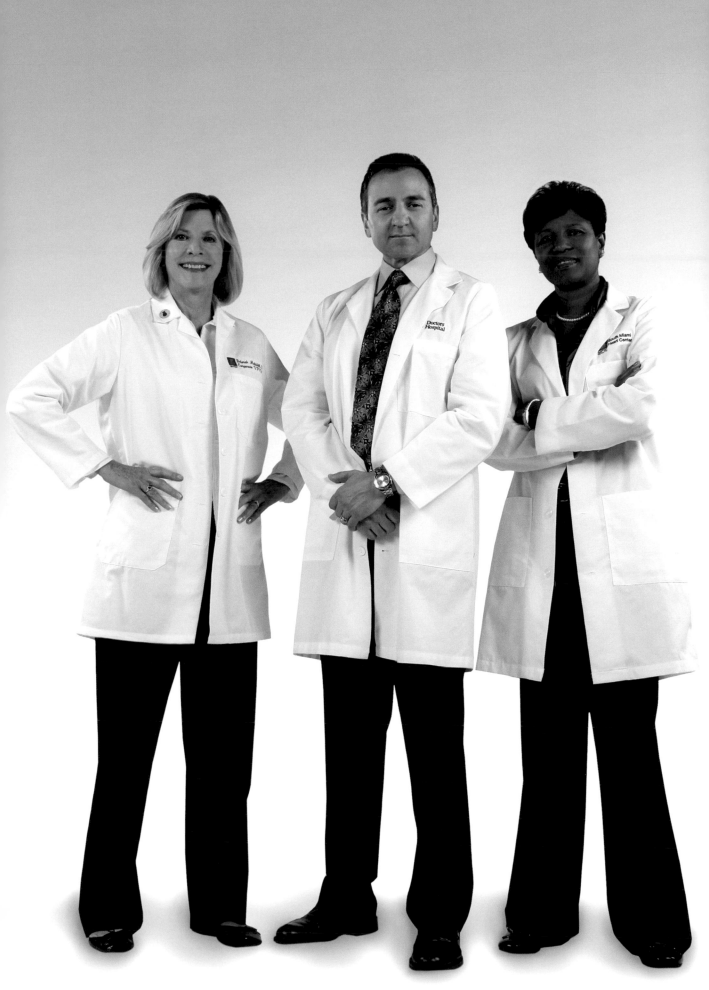

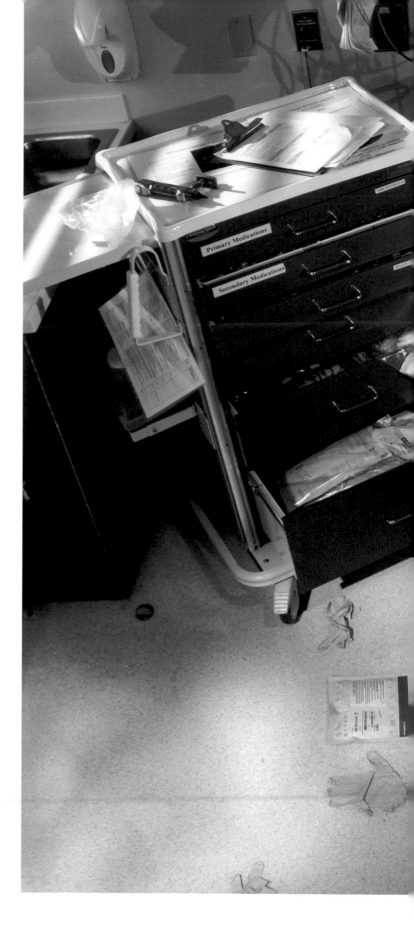

As nurses, we get very, very good at knowing when a patient is ready to die. Family members may not realize it, or they may have feelings of anger or guilt because they can't let go. Nurses are there to help them talk about it, to prepare them to say goodbye.

Because of our work, we can never get away from death. If you allow yourself to grieve and sympathize with patients and their families, it really gets to you. You have to keep yourself together and leave it behind at the end of the day, or you'll burn out very quickly.

SUSAN HOWARD, R.N.

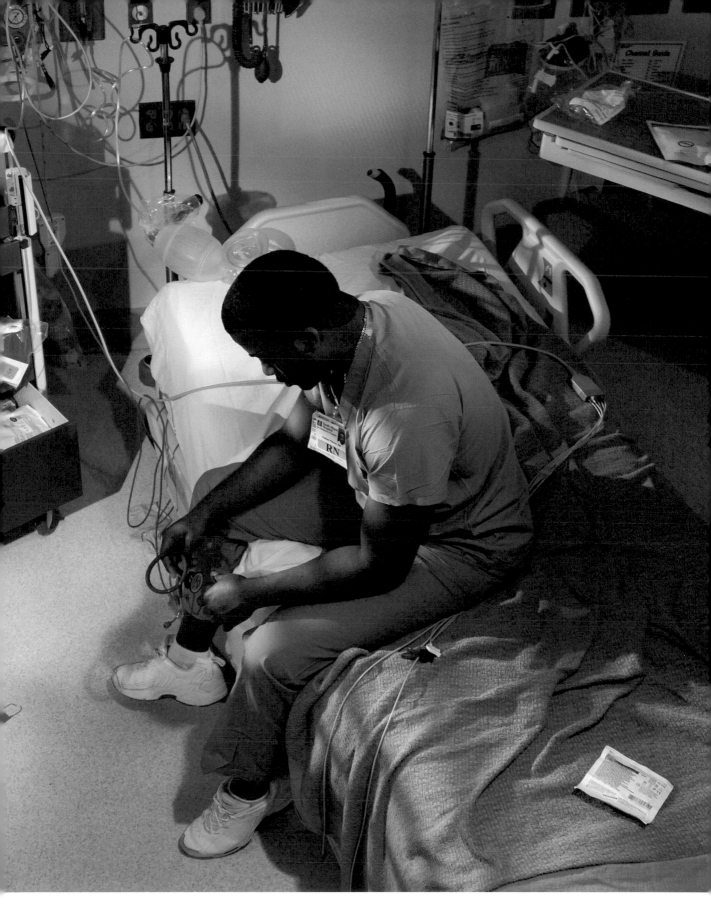

GRIEF

"Brilliance is so much more than an innate ability to understand nursing theory. Yes, you have to be smart, but you also have to apply the theory to each patient. It doesn't happen overnight; brilliance is something that evolves in a nurse. We develop a sixth sense."

MARIA SUAREZ, R.N.

BRILLIANCE

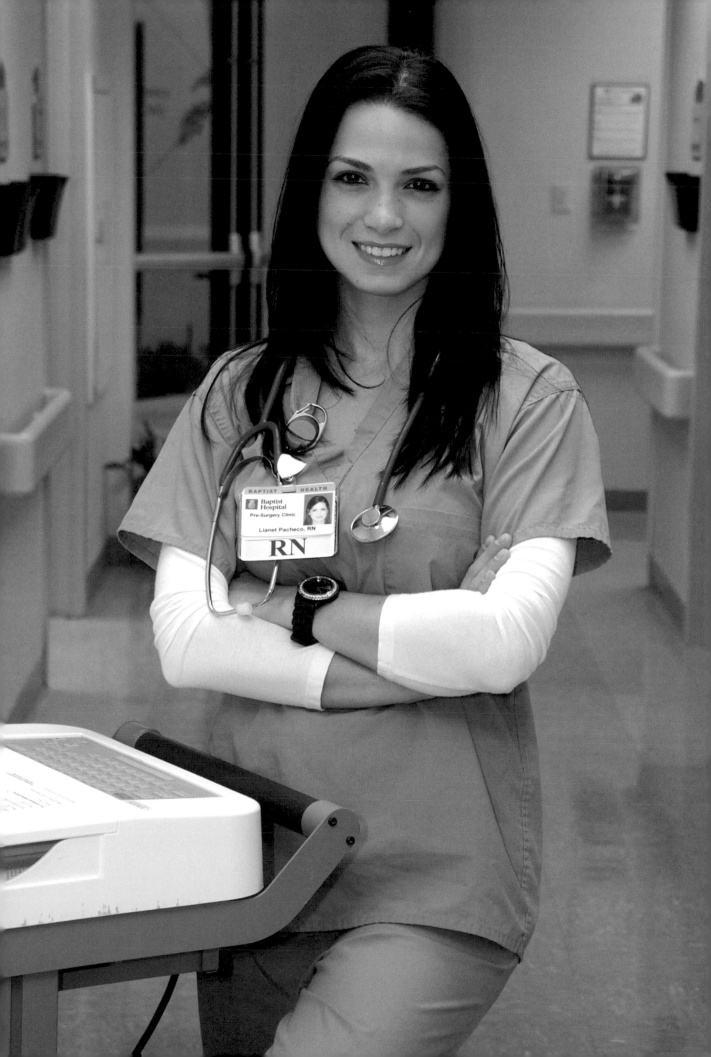

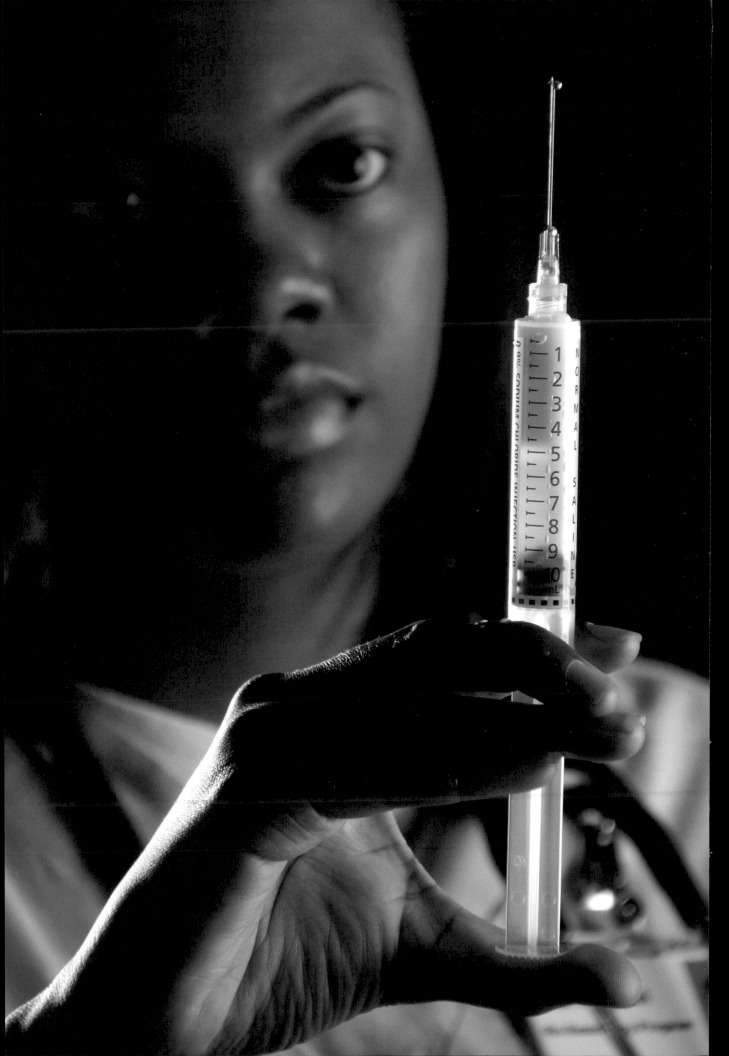

" No nurse ever has just one 'job'. While we keep our eye on the current task or assignment, we know that we'll have something else to attend to immediately afterward. The best nurses never lose sight of the fact that our job exists for the sake of the best patient care, treatment and service. We constantly strive for success, even when we hit a roadblock. "

CHERYL BROWN, R.N.

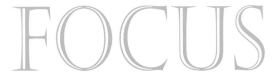

FOCUS

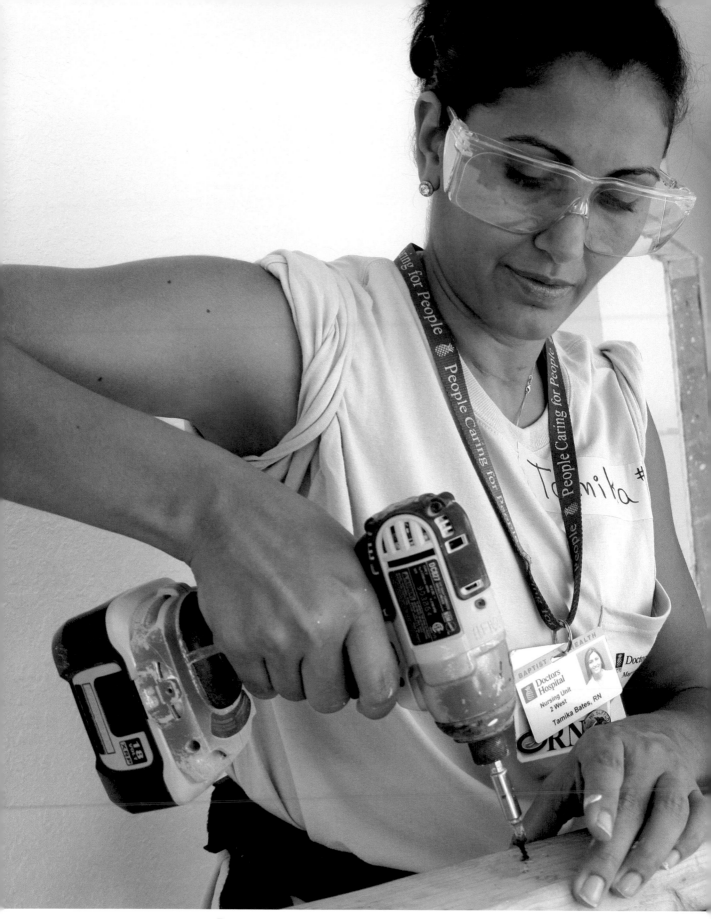

SERVICE

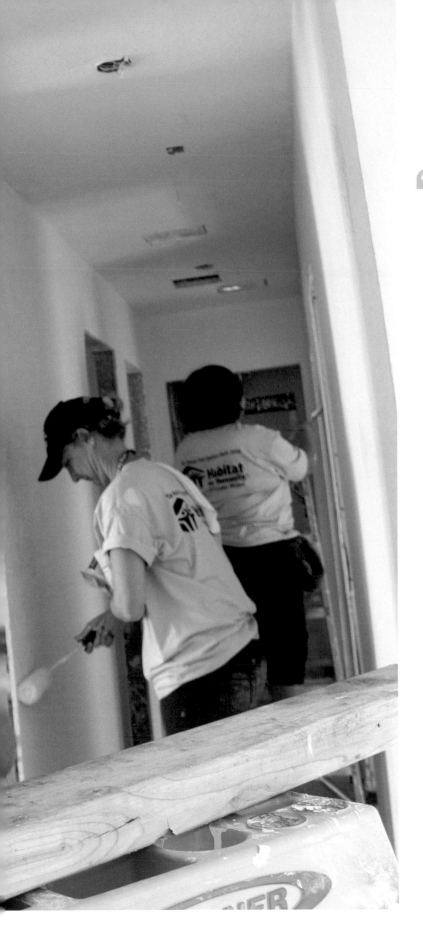

> " *To me, service means treating every patient the way I or my family members would want to be treated. It's more than just what we do; it's the way we do it. Our behavior as nurses needs to express the genuine attitude that this patient is the only patient, and we will do whatever it takes to ensure that the best care is given.* "

SANDY HYATT, R.N.

characterized by ardent dedication and loyalty…

DEVOTED

" Healthcare professionals respect one another as team members. Knowing you are respected gives you confidence and makes you want to do a better job.

I have seen the role of the nurse change so much. It used to be that we just carried out the instructions of the physician. Now, physicians acknowledge the amount of personal time we spend with patients and listen to our recommendations regarding treatment. We are rightly viewed as important members of the care team. "

LAURA COSLER, R.N.

RESPECT

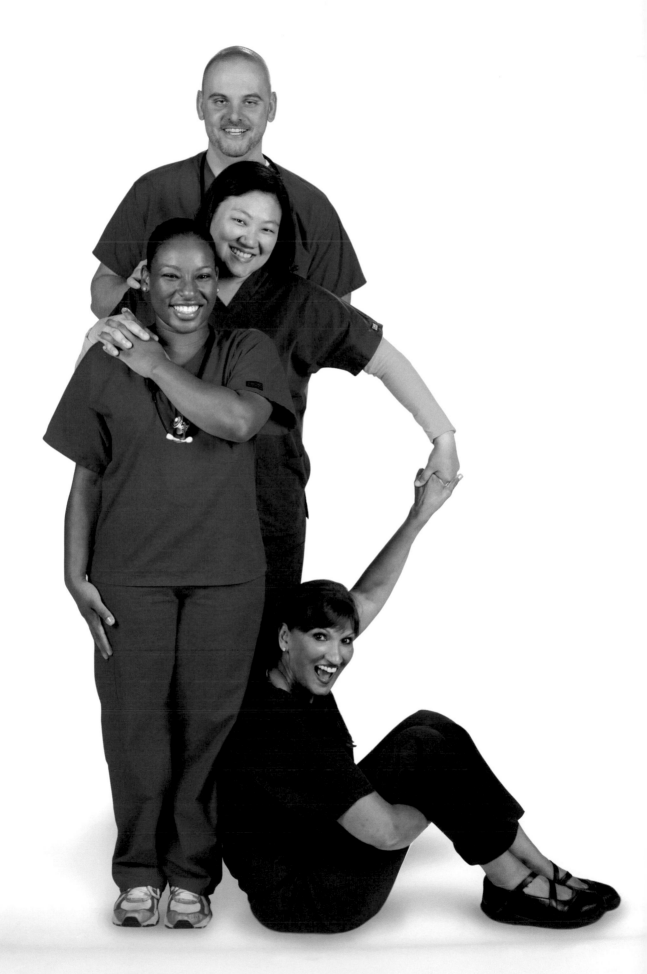

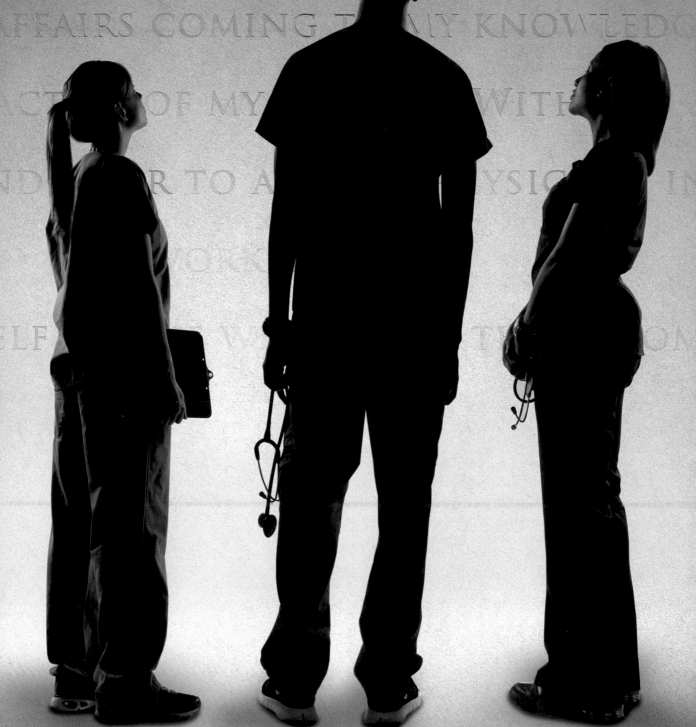

"Nurses have clear ethical standards, guidelines and principles. When we become nurses, we become an advocate for the patient's health, safety and rights, which means we must operate according to the patient's and family's values while assuring the most positive outcome. We have to remember we are here to serve the patient, regardless of who they are or what they believe in."

ROSE ALLEN, R.N.

ETHICS

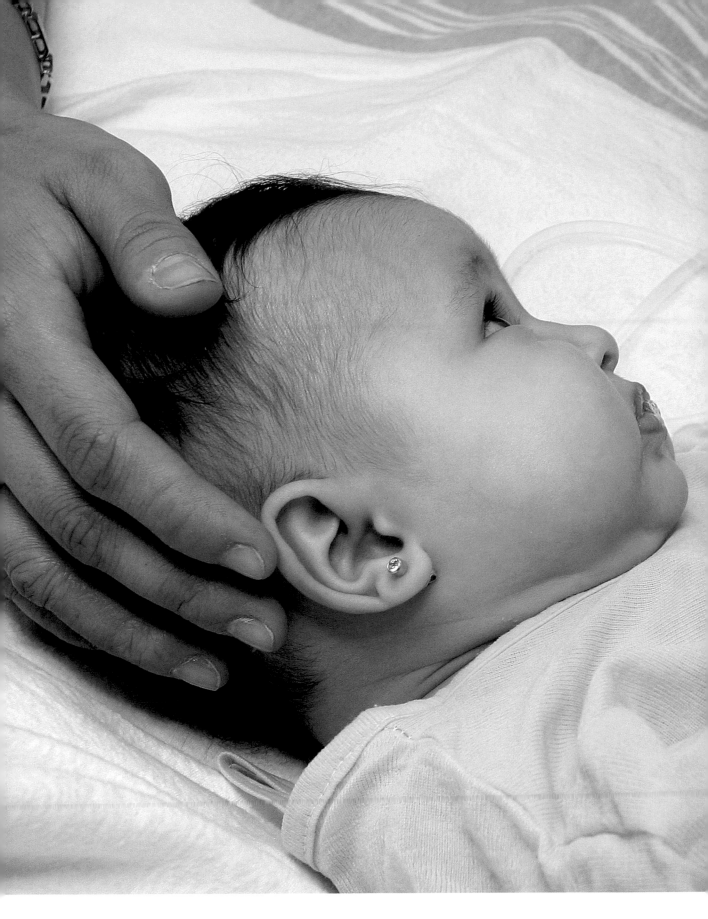

INTEGRITY

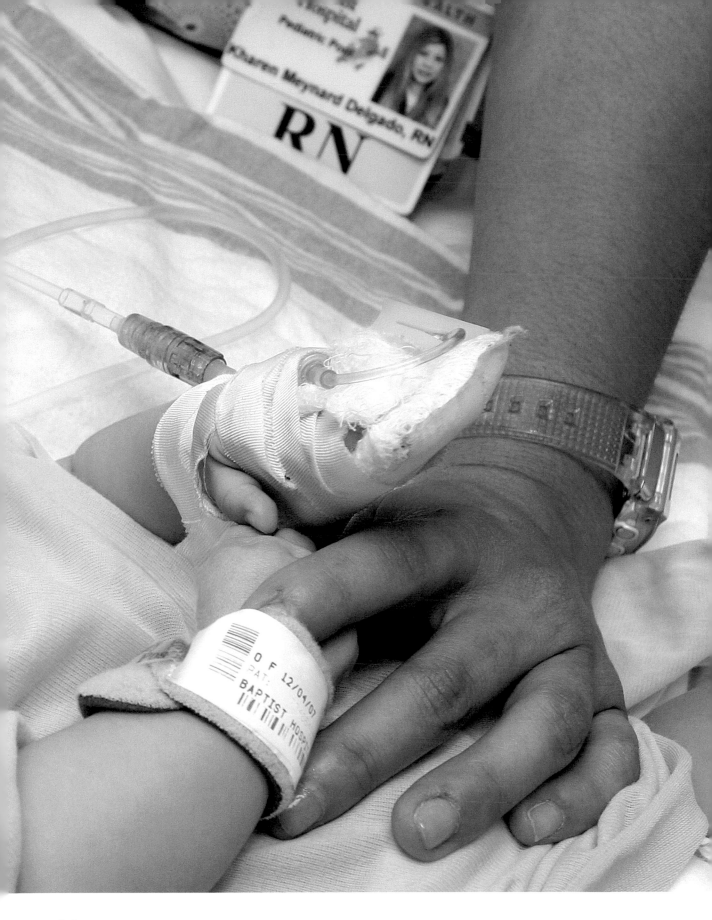

❝ *People who are hospitalized with an injury or illness are at their most vulnerable. They seem to know instinctively that they need to put their trust in someone who will take responsibility for their care, and that someone is always the nurse.* **❞**

LOURDES CASTANEDA-JACOBS, R.N.

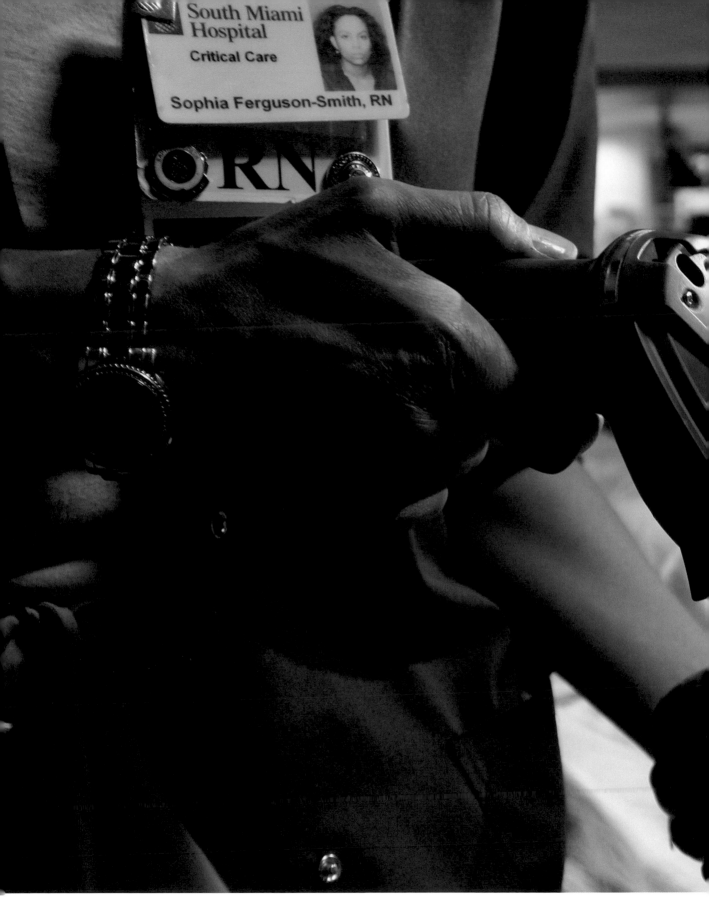

“ *Nurses are committed to doing the very best they can every day, with concern, compassion and care for every patient. One error can be devastating to both the patient and the staff. We strive to learn from every mistake and share that knowledge not only within our own hospitals, but nationwide.* ”

GERI SCHIMMEL, R.N.

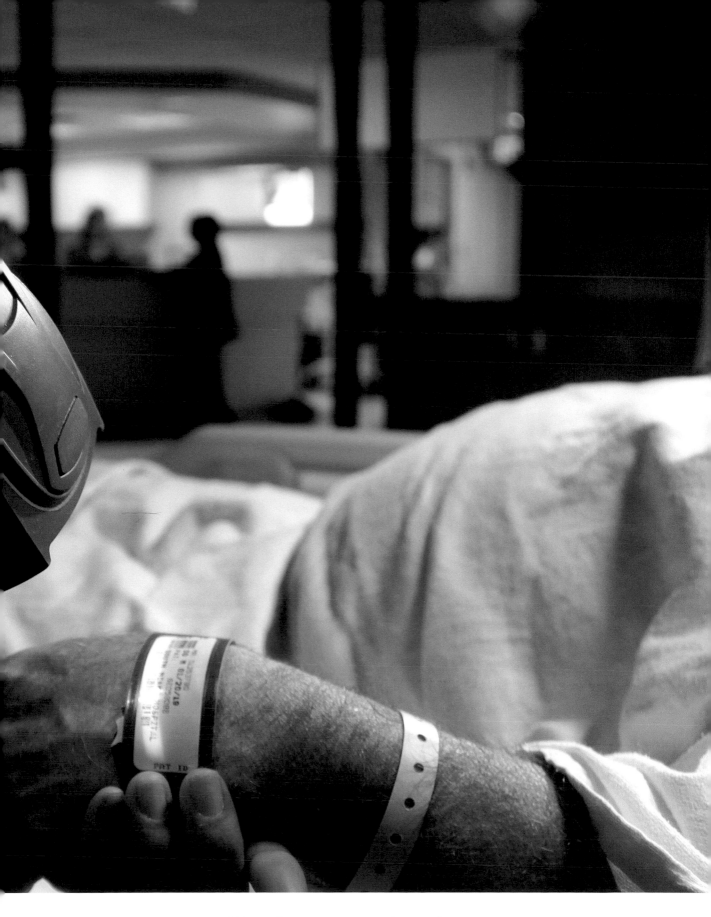

SAFETY

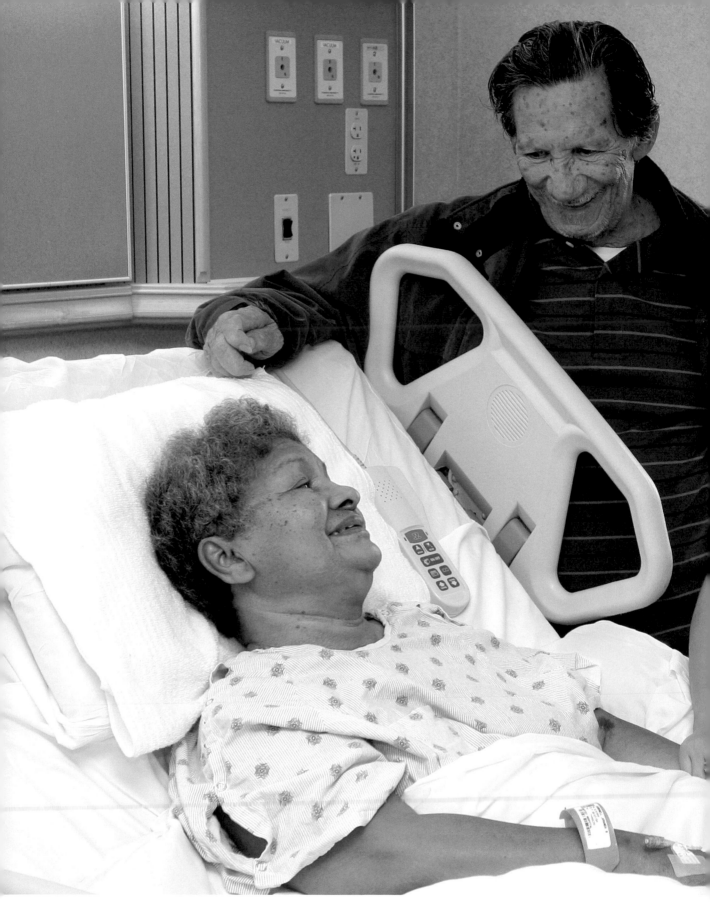

PATIENT- AND FAMILY-

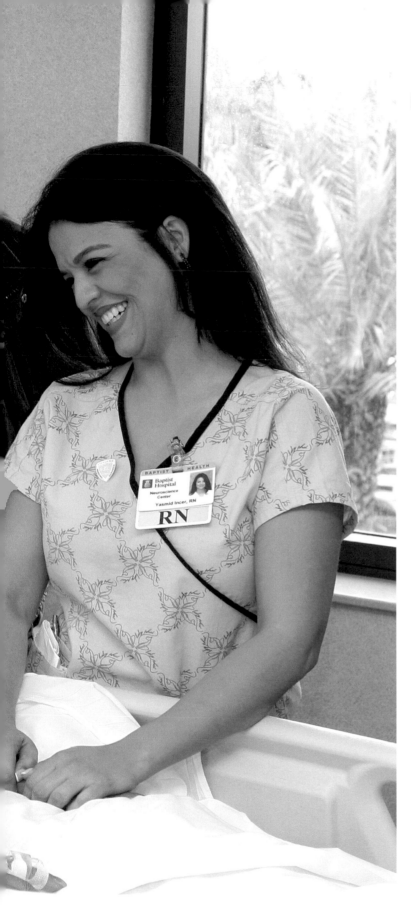

"Medicine has shifted from a 'we know best' attitude to a more collaborative approach with patients and their families. We understand that they must be our partners in the process of healthcare delivery.

Patient- and family-centered care begins with listening to the voice of the patient. Family members also can help us pick up on small nuances; for example, a mother may know exactly how to interpret her toddler's babbling. When an elderly patient loses his aspect, his child may understand what his facial expressions mean.

This more engaged style of care is not any more time-consuming, yet supports better outcomes as well as improved patient satisfaction."

DENISE HARRIS, R.N.

CENTERED CARE

*marked
by deep
understanding
and sound
judgment...*

WISE

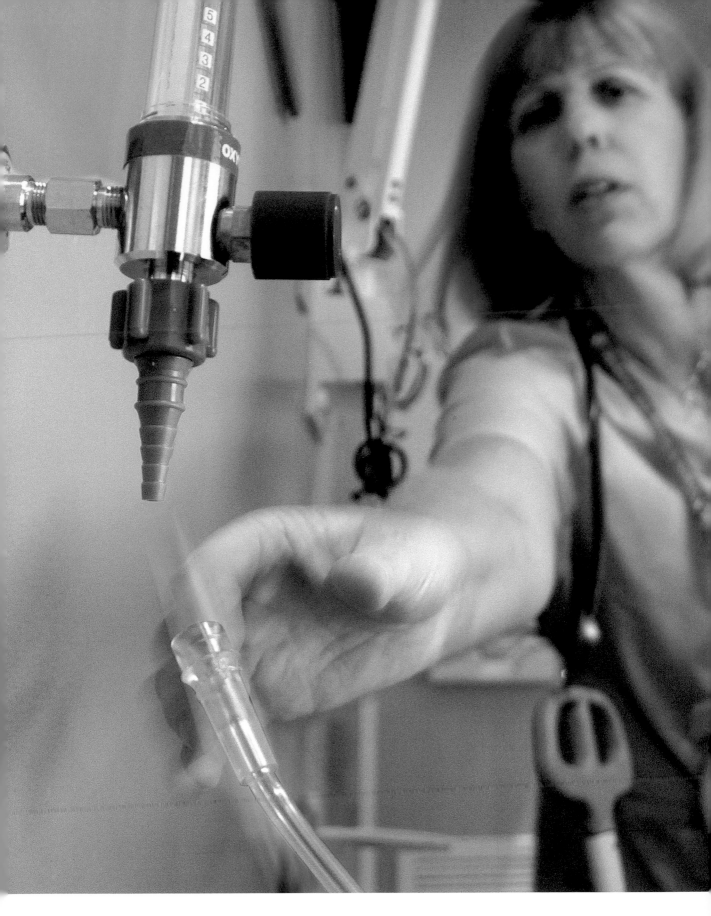

PERCEPTION

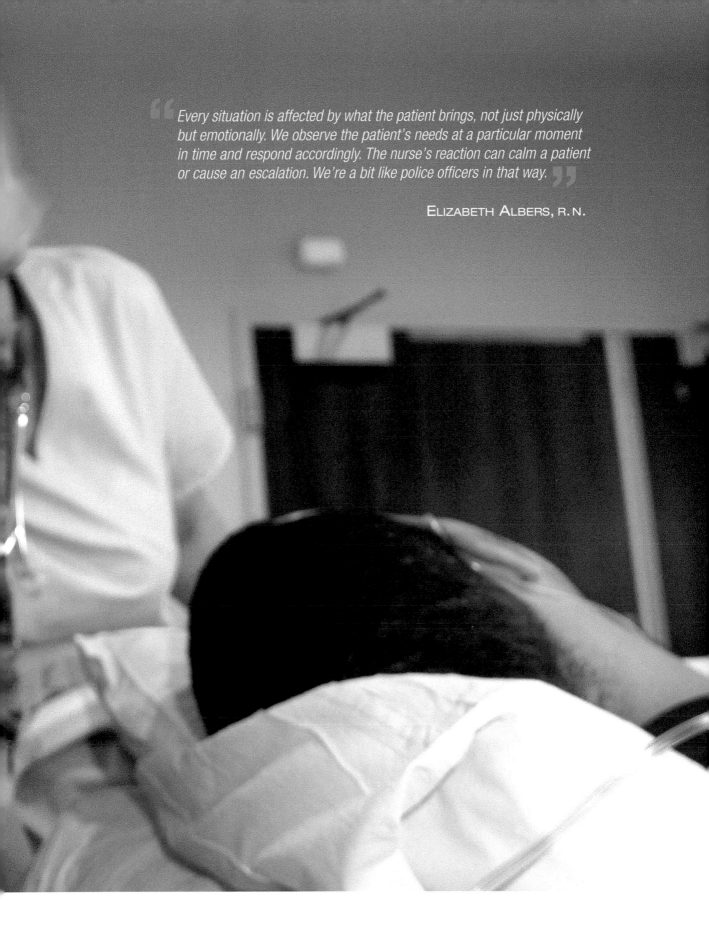

"Every situation is affected by what the patient brings, not just physically but emotionally. We observe the patient's needs at a particular moment in time and respond accordingly. The nurse's reaction can calm a patient or cause an escalation. We're a bit like police officers in that way."

ELIZABETH ALBERS, R.N.

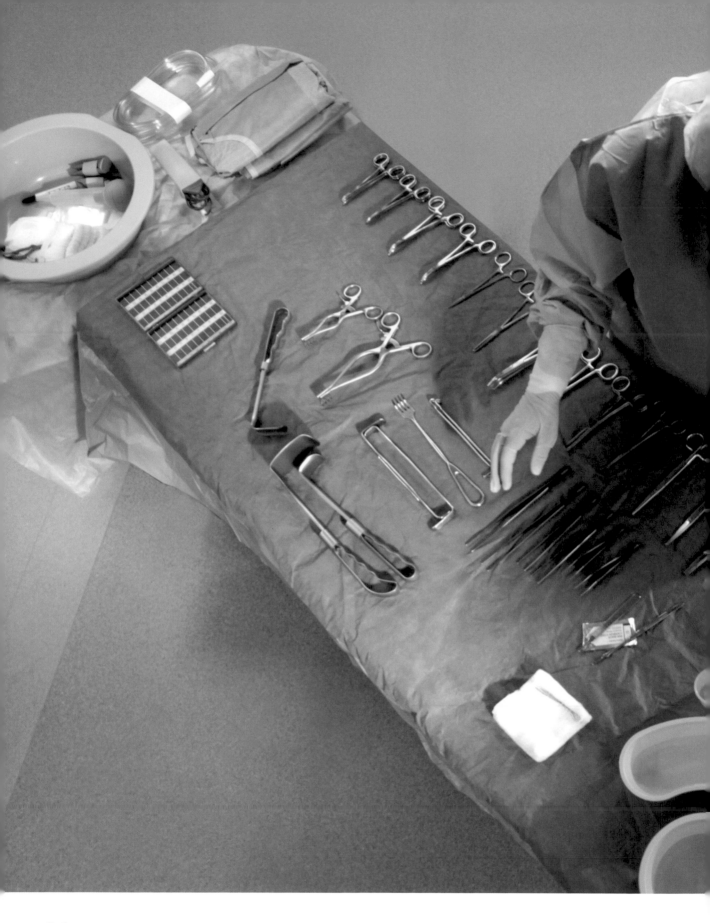

It's a good feeling to say, at the end of the day, 'I did everything possible, based on everything I know.' Accuracy comes from learning continually and being engaged 100 percent in what you're doing.

DEBBIE SMITH, R.N.

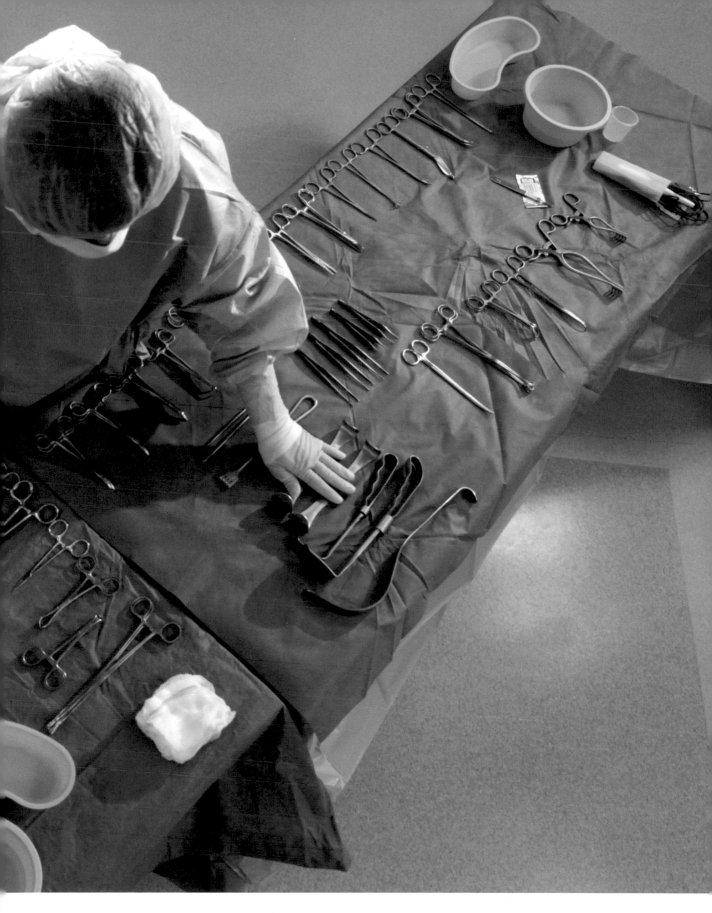

ACCURACY

"*Every morning I ask myself, 'Am I prepared for the challenges I will face in the next eight to 12 hours?' As nurses, we recommit ourselves daily to our calling as caregivers. We persevere.*"

KATHERINE TRYON, R.N.

DEDICATION

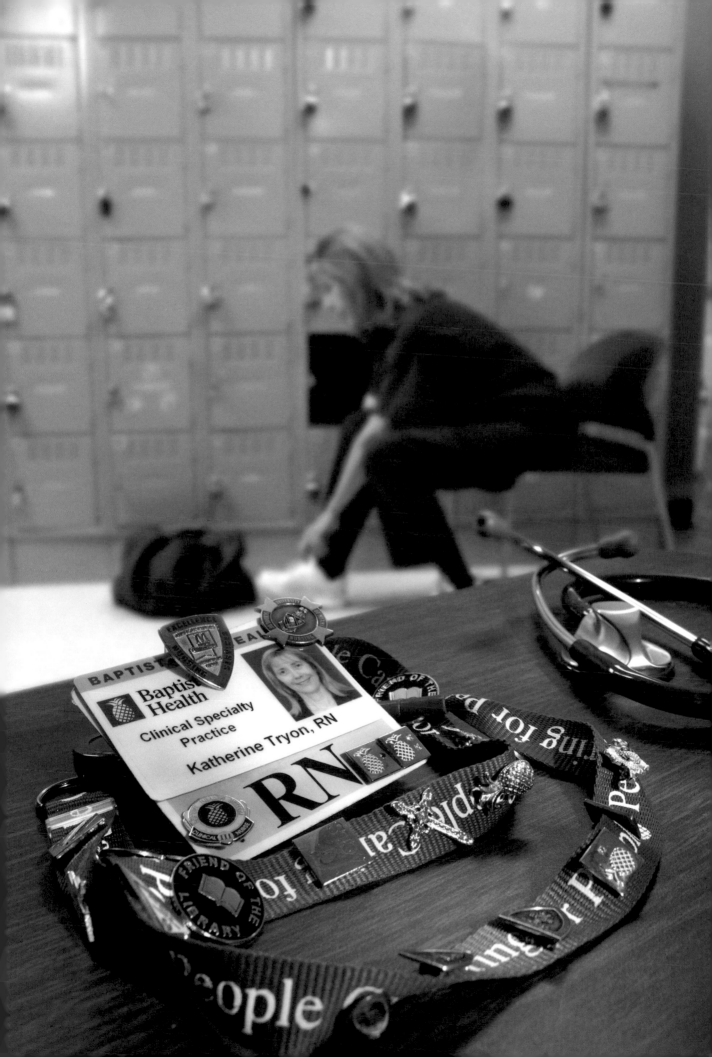

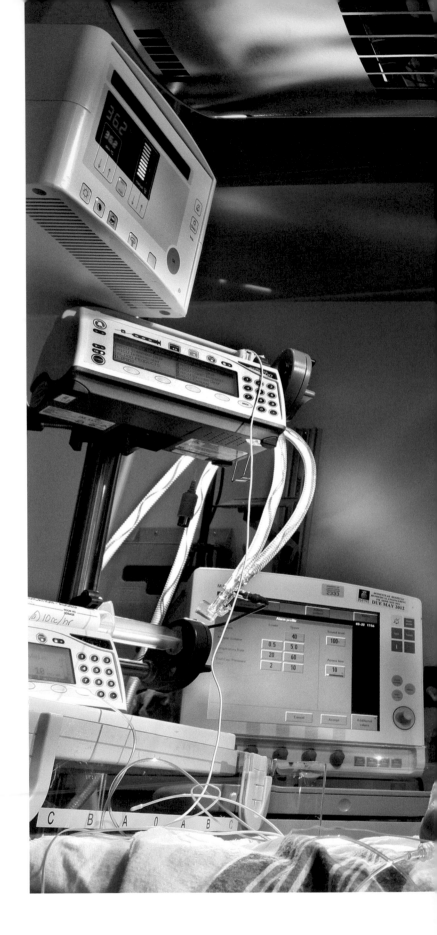

“ *The public's expectations of their healthcare experience are greater than ever. Nurses are encouraged to study for that extra degree or certification to stay competitive in their field. But, competency is more than just knowledge — it also grows from the critical thinking skills that develop from hands-on patient care. Competency is empowering. It drives me to go further and learn more.* ”

NANCY MARTINEZ, R.N.

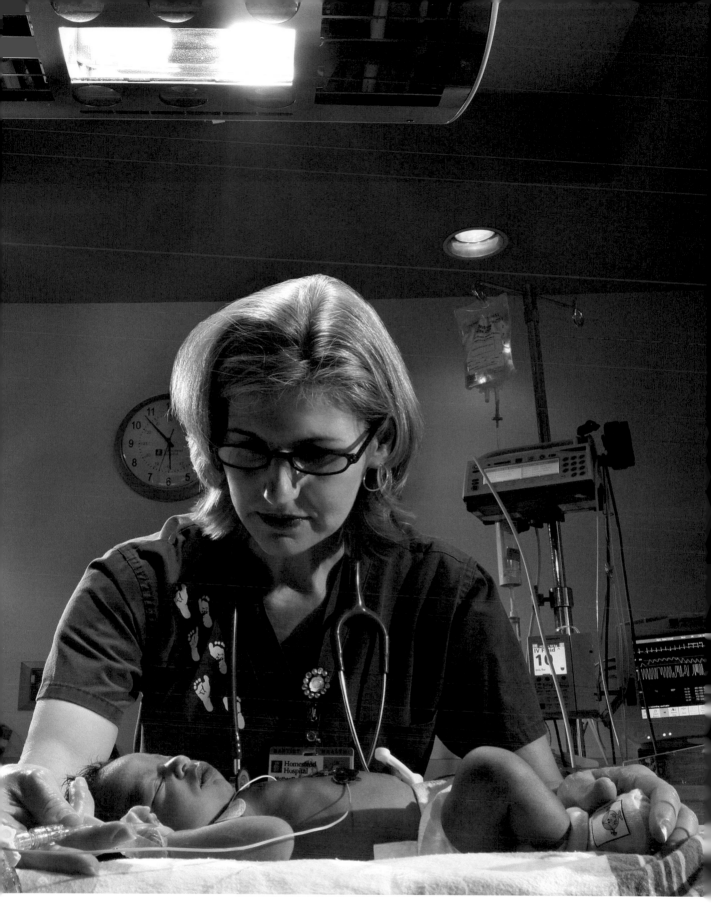

COMPETENCE

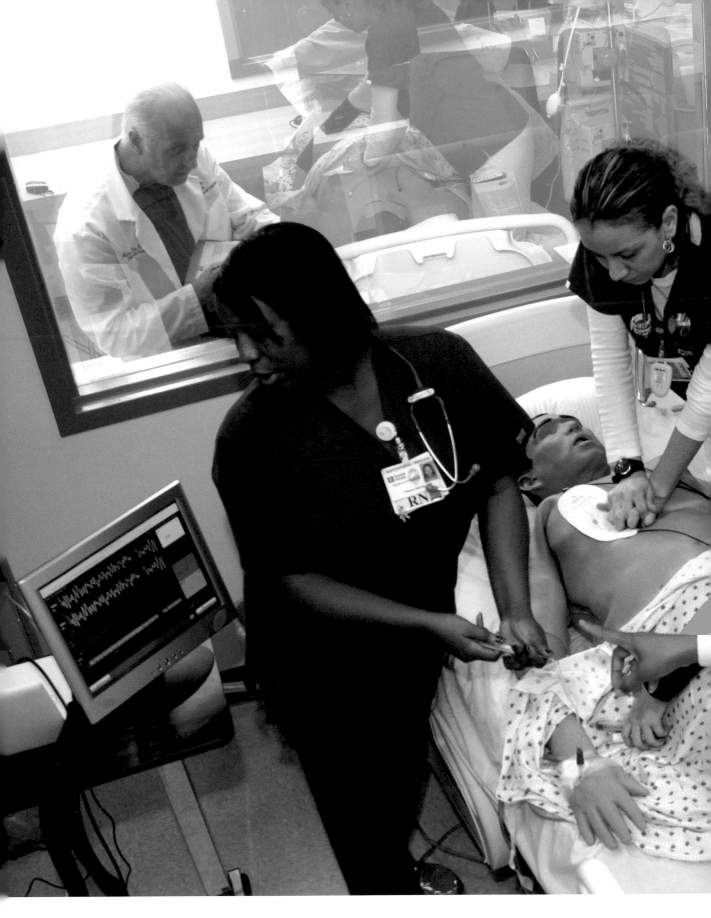

KNOWLEDGE

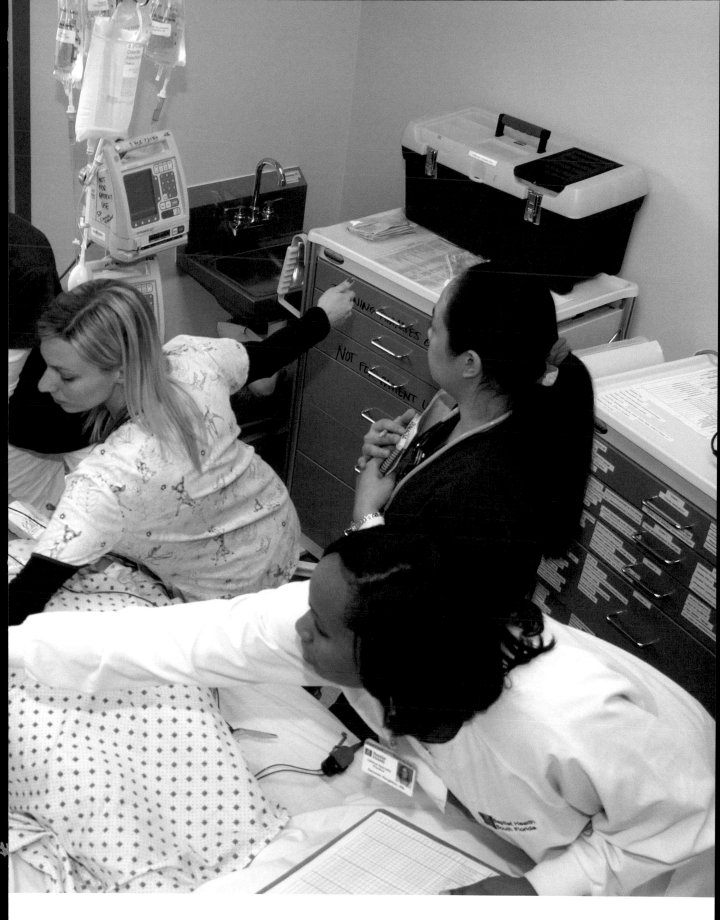

> Each of us brings something to the table — it's just a matter of identifying it and making it happen. Every situation presents an opportunity to learn something and pass it on. The first step is asking, 'What can I do to make a difference?'

PATRICIA RONQUILLO, R.N.

*bound by
a pledge
or an*

assurance...

COMMITTED

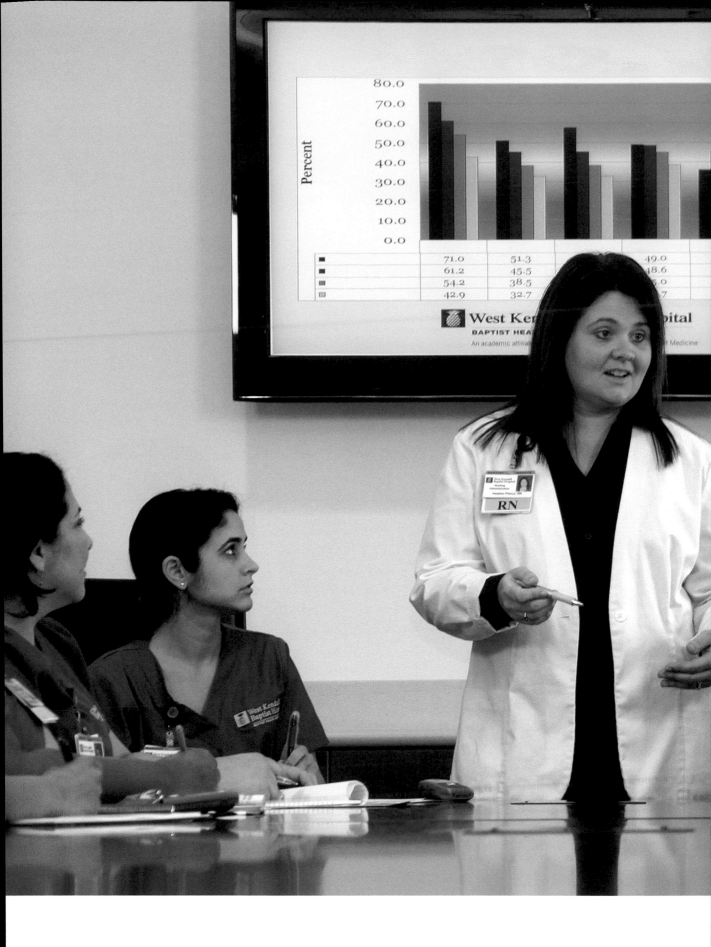

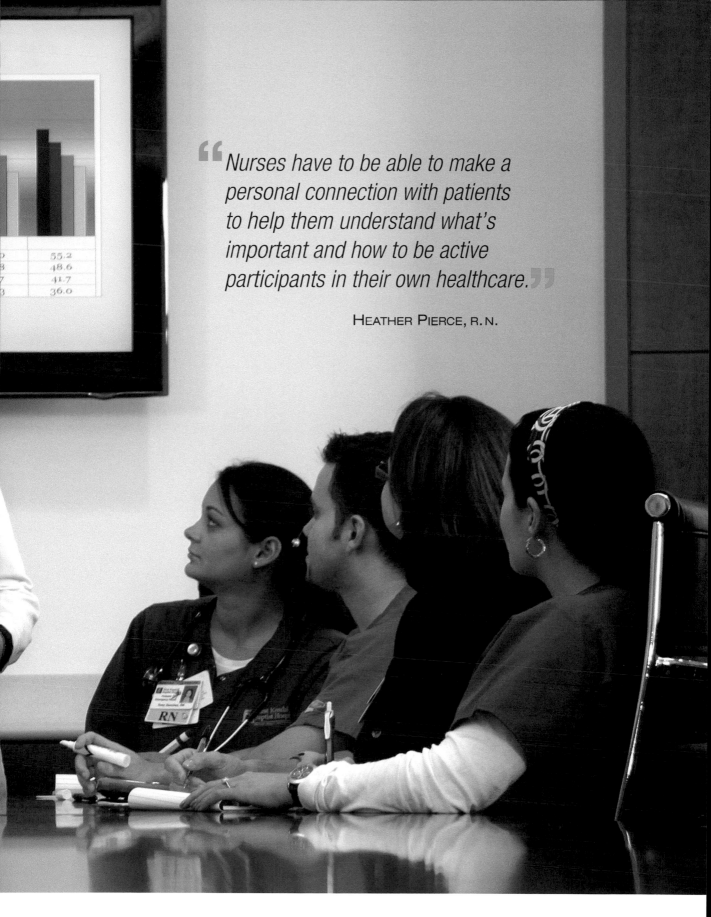

> *"Nurses have to be able to make a personal connection with patients to help them understand what's important and how to be active participants in their own healthcare."*
>
> HEATHER PIERCE, R.N.

ENGAGEMENT

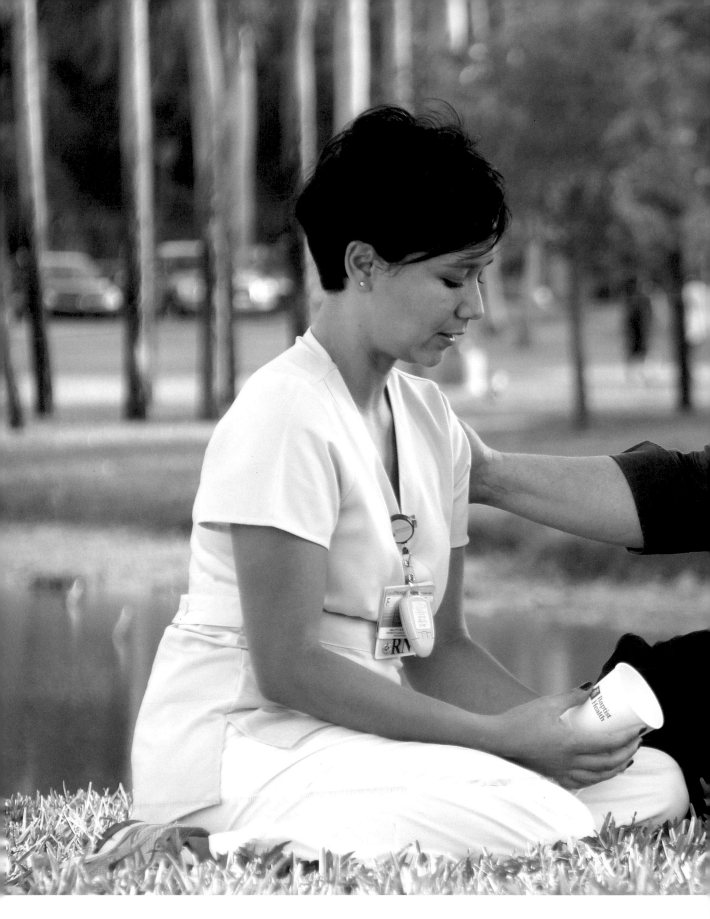

MENTORSHIP

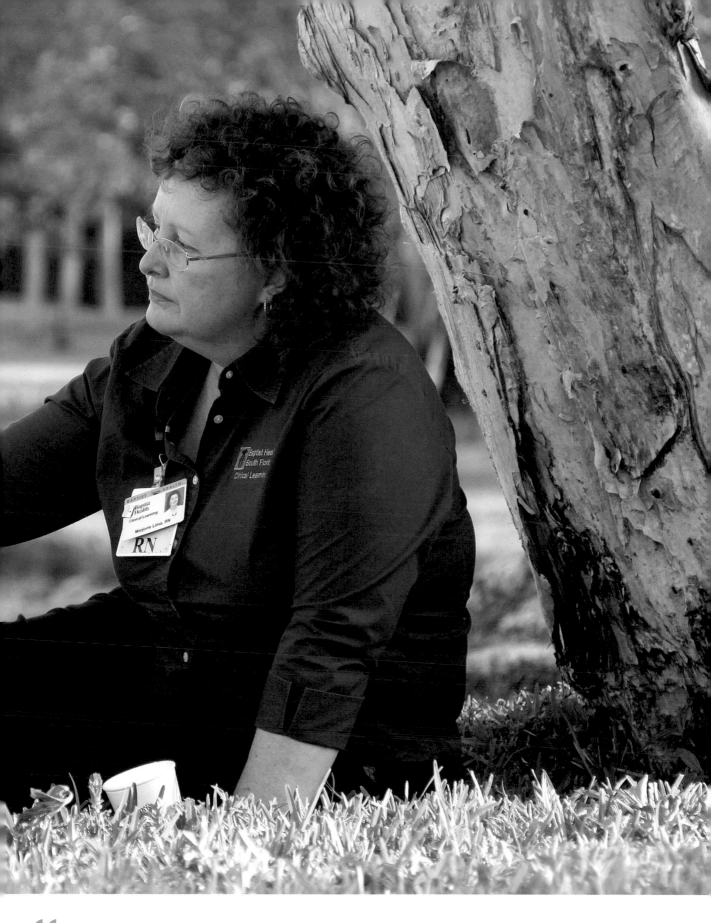

"*All new nurses should look seriously at finding someone to help guide their career. People who have had a mentor seem to have better mechanisms for coping and making decisions. It's so useful to have an objective and knowledgeable person to turn to for advice.*"

MARJORIE LIMA, R.N.

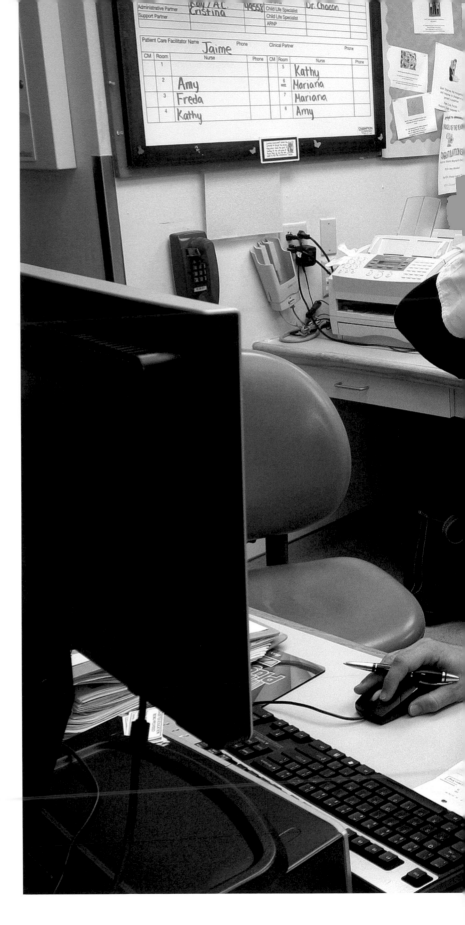

> " While physicians closely follow a patient's progress, nurses are available to the patient constantly. We develop a plan of care for the patient and interact with all of the other disciplines as they are called in. The nurse is at the center of it all; we can't delegate that. "

MILLY SELGAS, R.N.

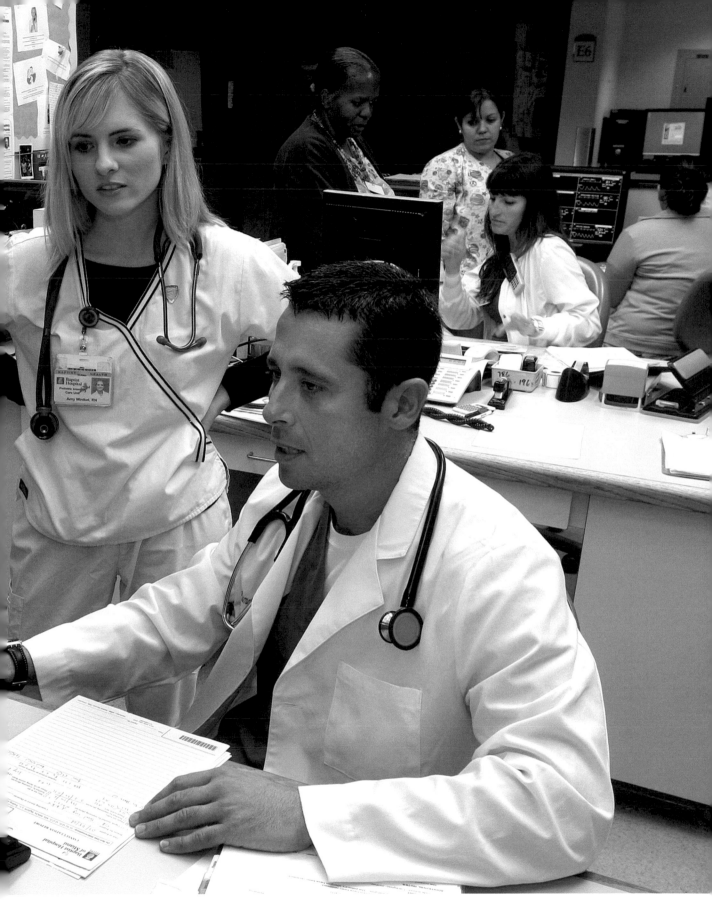

COLLABORATION

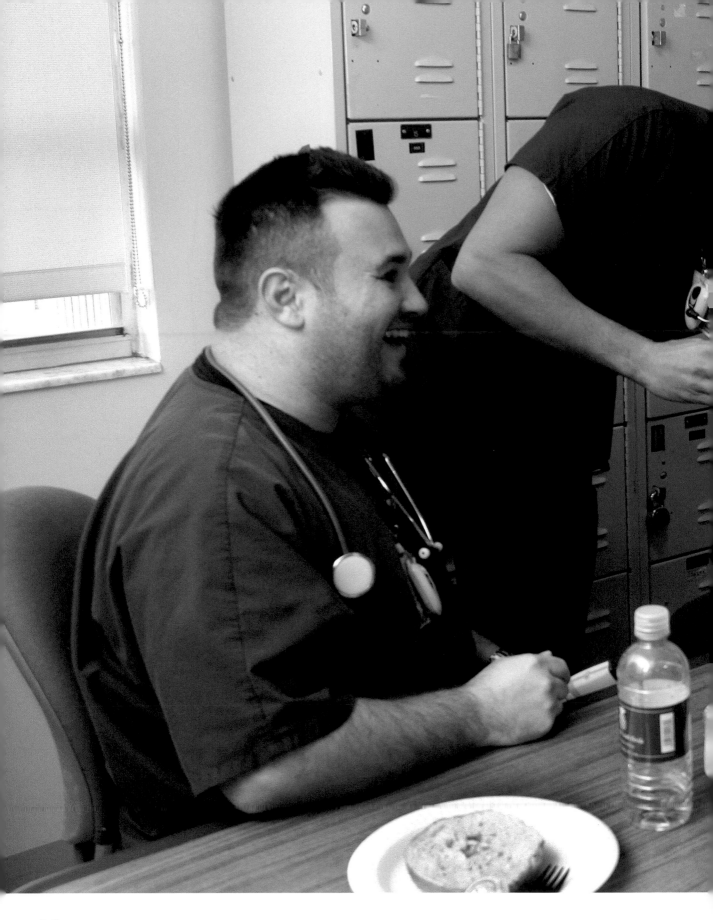

“ *Nurses wear so many hats these days — one day I'm a manager, the next day I'm bathing a patient. We rely on each other and on other departments so much. I'm confident that regardless of the situation, I can call on any member of the care team and know they would be there for me.* ”

DEBRA STANGER, R.N.

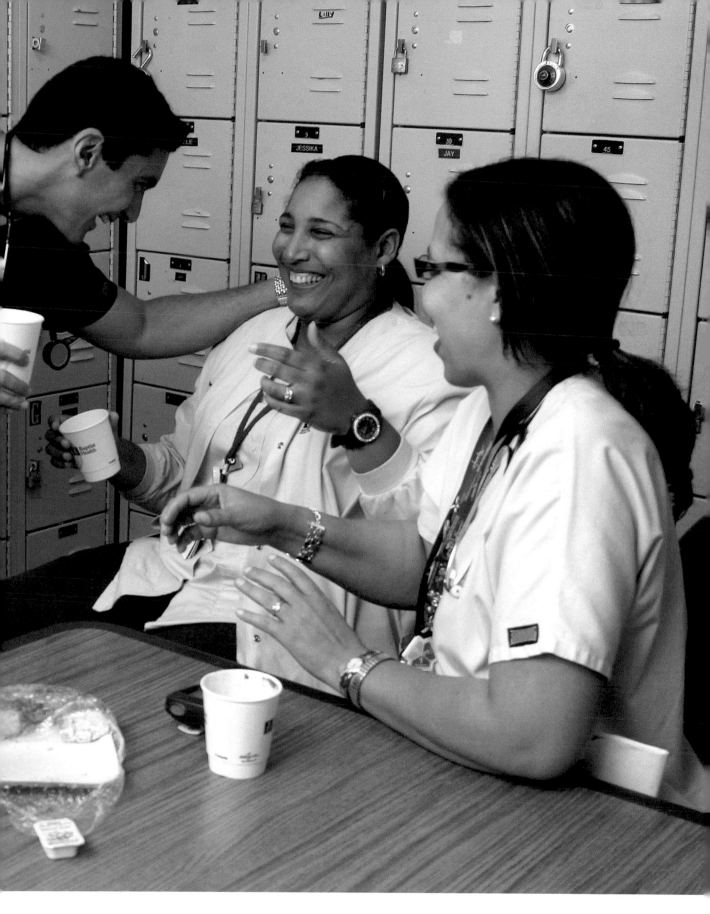

CAMARADERIE

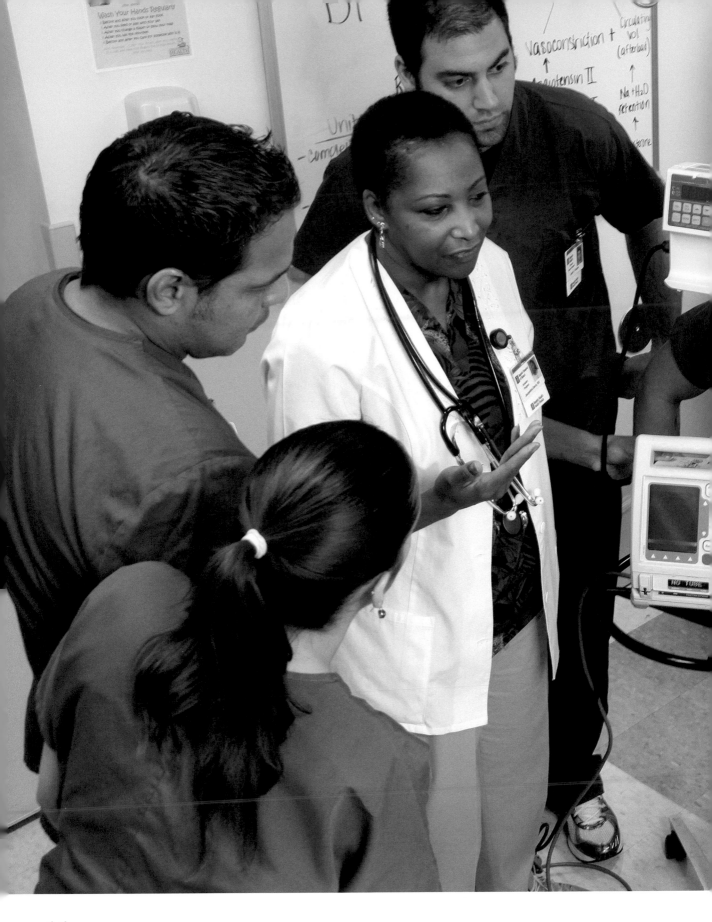

> Technology is advancing so rapidly that we have to work hard to keep our skills up to date. As a professional educator, I feel a tremendous obligation to share my knowledge with other nurses. In addition to teaching clinical skills, we immerse our nurses in a culture of nurturing and caring.

JACQUELINE DAVIS, R.N.

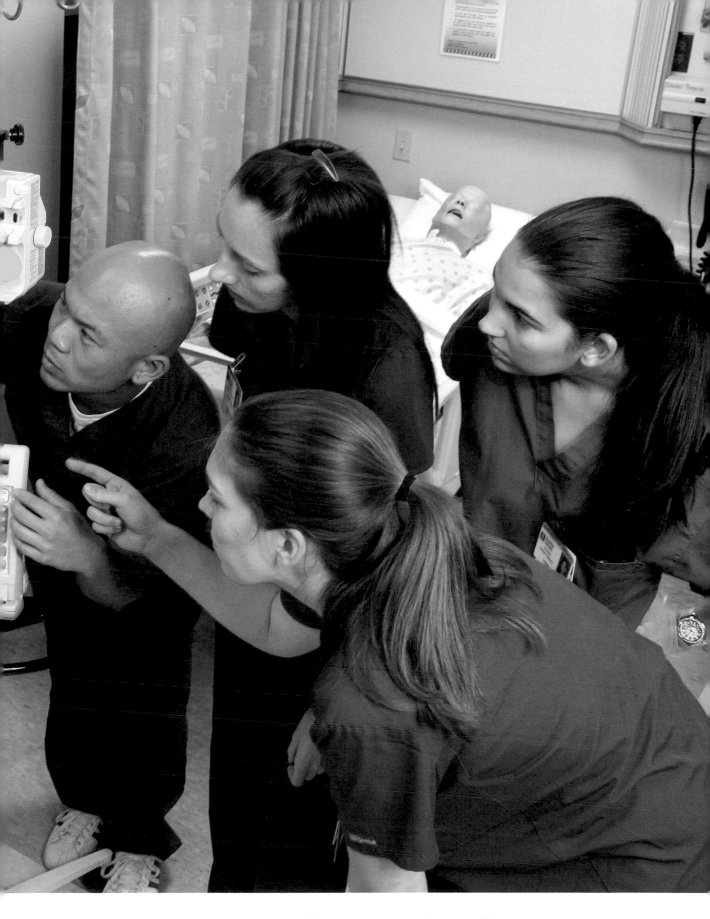

EDUCATION

deviating from the norm, better than average...

EXCEPTIONAL

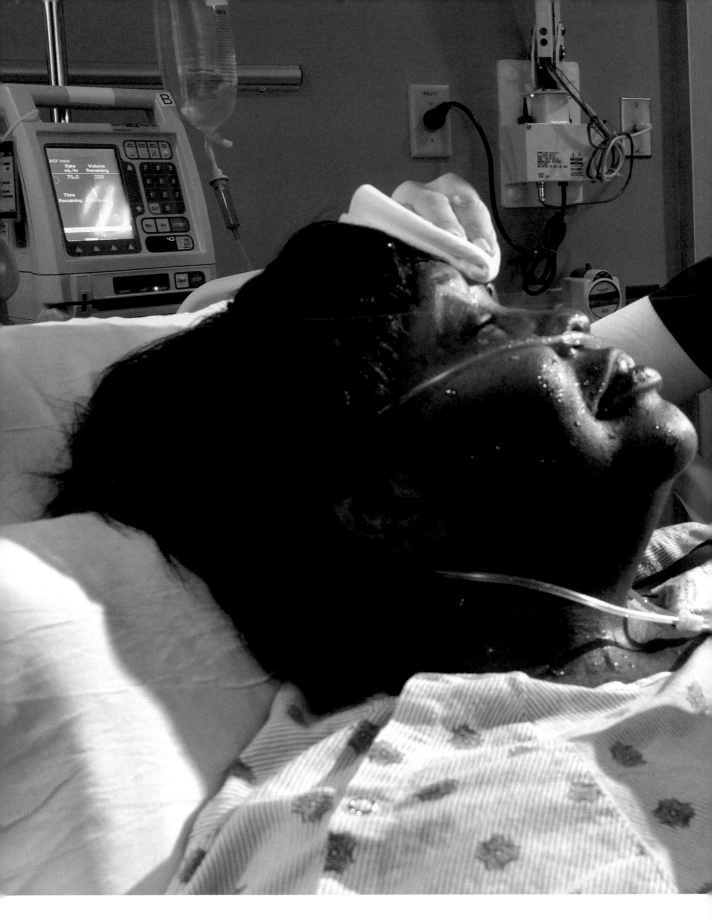

EMPATHY

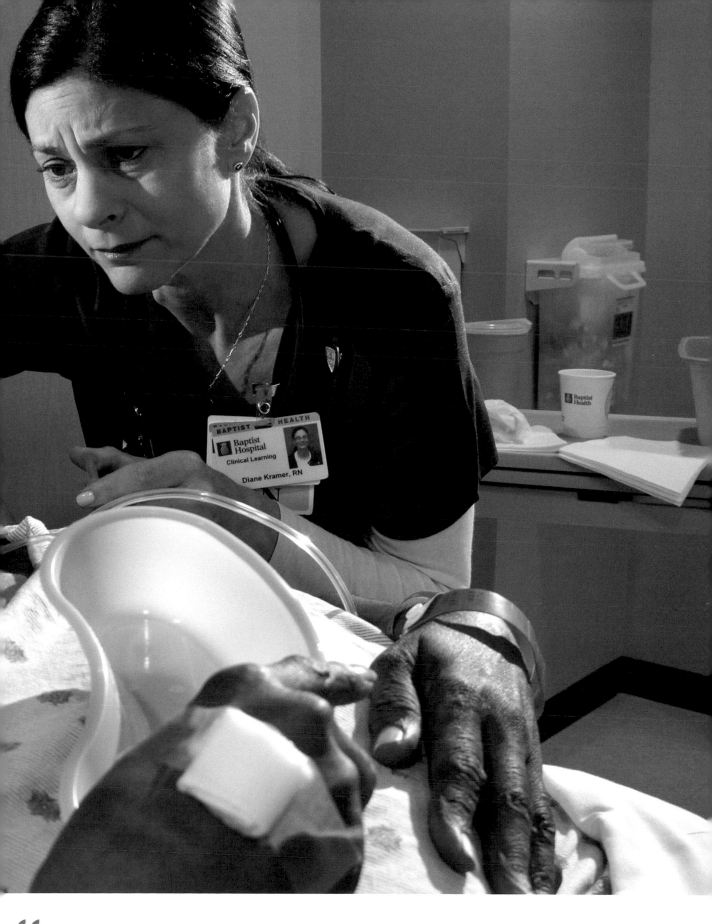

"I think of empathy as being able to identify with the pain others are experiencing in a particular moment. Some nurses can identify too closely, to the point that it becomes an emotional drain. The wonderful thing about the profession is that nurses understand what their colleagues are going through and are there to provide support."

CHAPLAIN RONALD GAUDIO

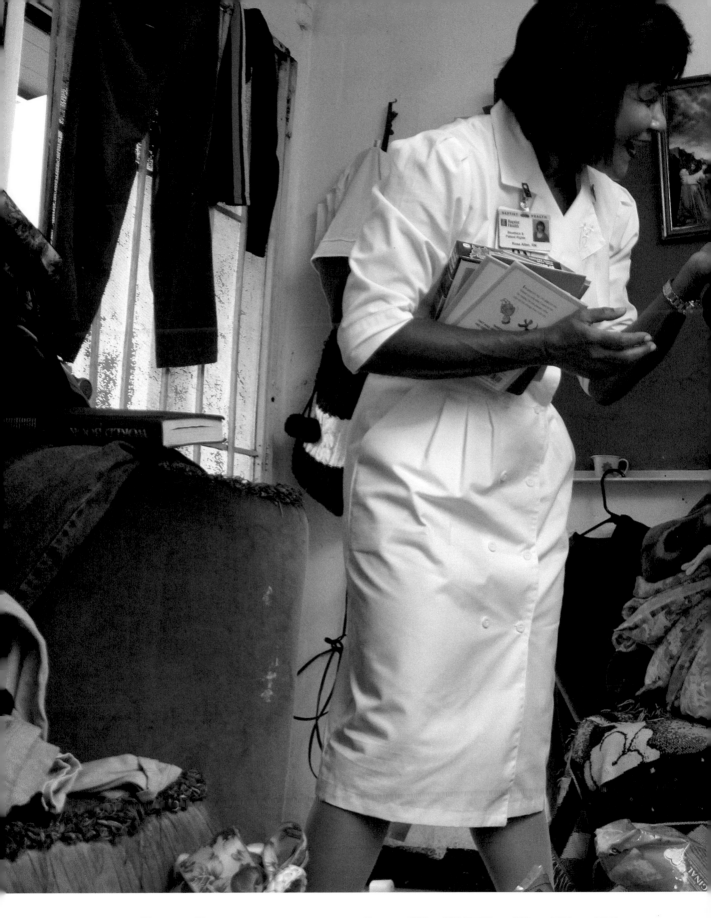

COMPASSION

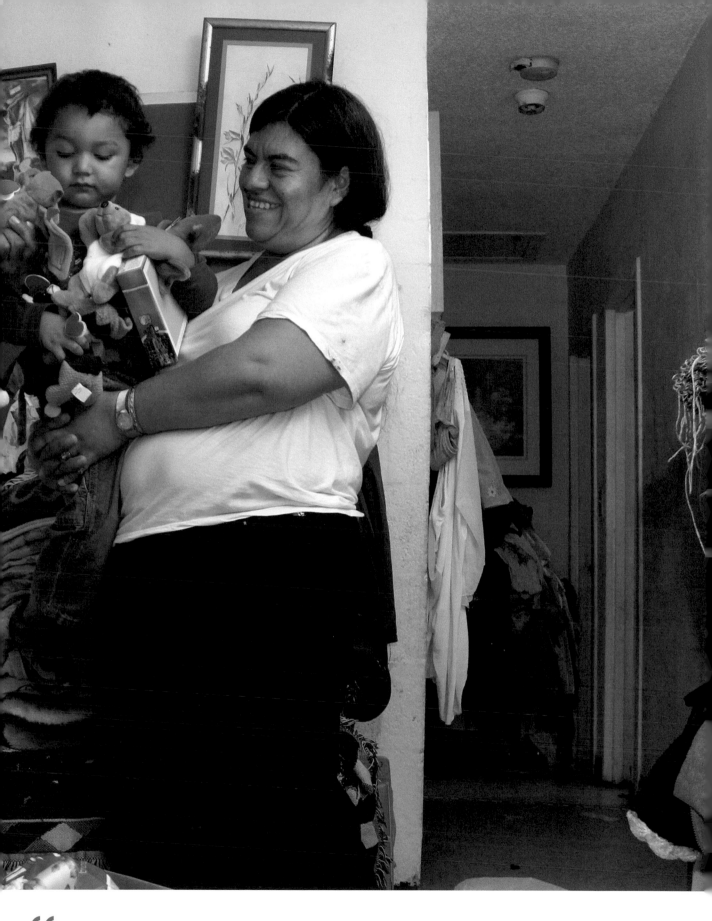

"When infants and children are sick, nurses connect with moms and dads to help them understand what they are going through. In a way, we become part of their family. The most rewarding experience is when we discharge a patient; it's wonderful to help a sick child finally get home."

MARIA OLMEDA, R.N.

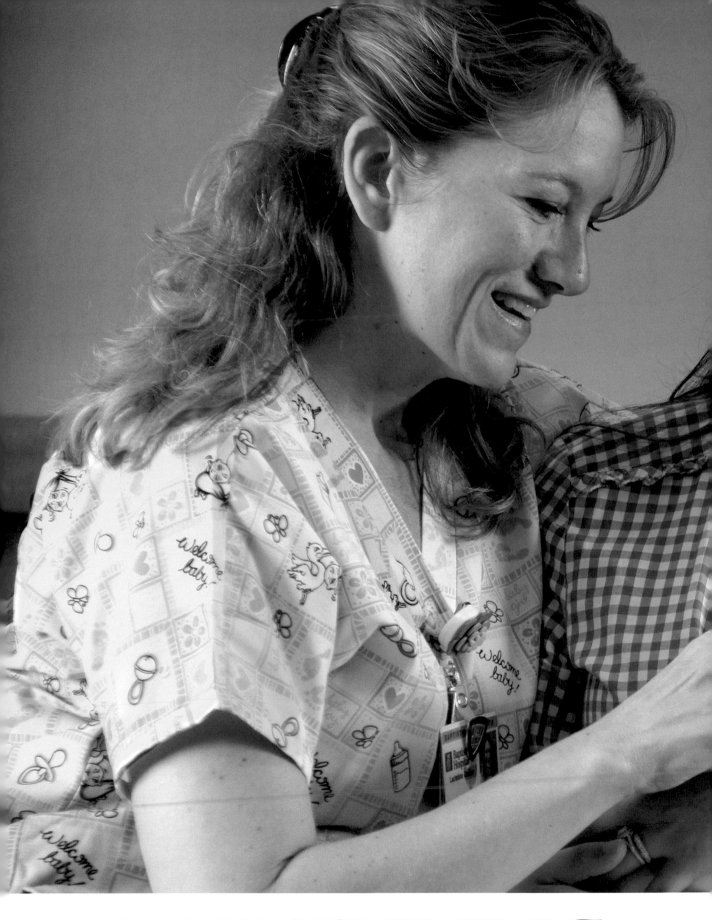

NURTURING

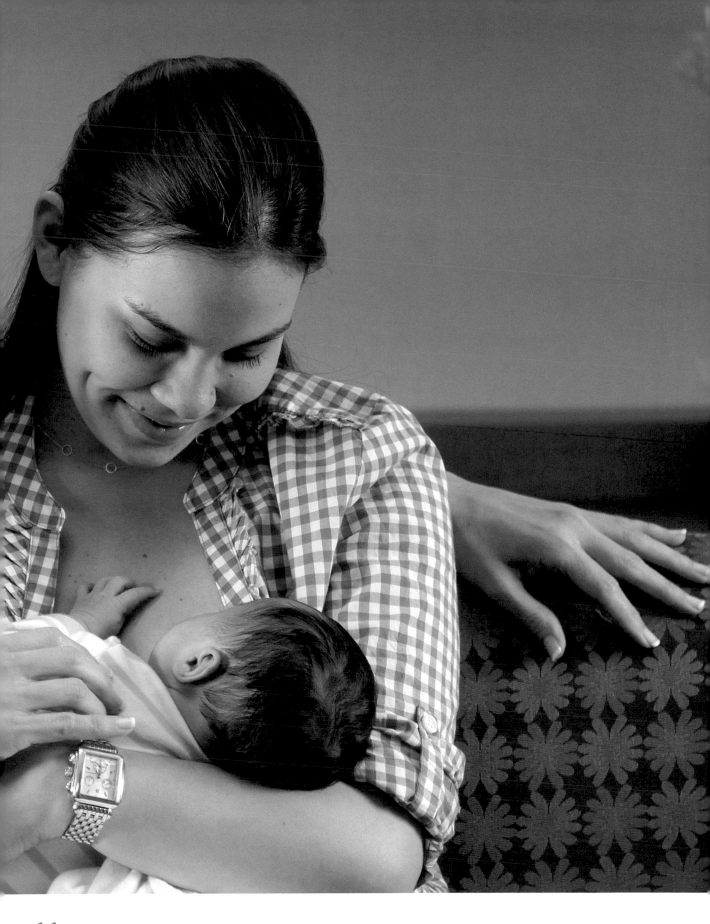

" Nurturing is the basis of the nurse-patient relationship, but it is also critical to the relationship between nurses. We take care to foster new nurses, particularly those who are new graduates, in an atmosphere that builds their confidence and brings out their own nurturing side. "

JOSE GUITIAN, R.N.

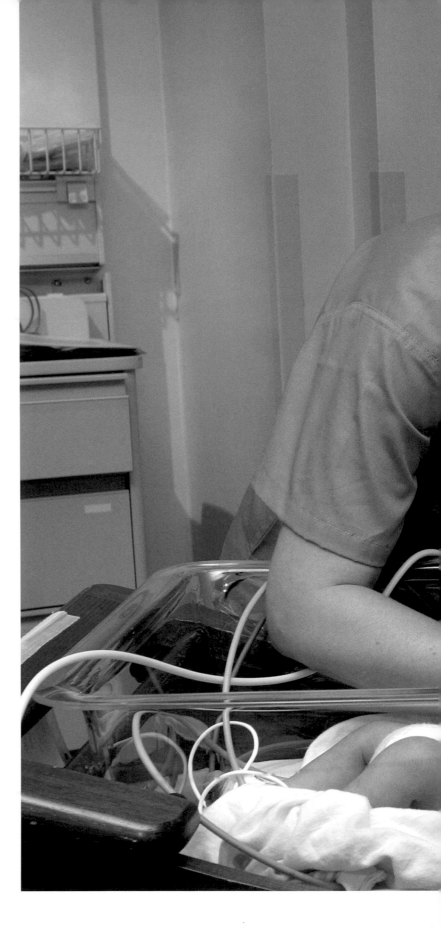

"Caring for a sick child sometimes feels like treating three patients — the child plus the mother and father. Kids are fun. They want to play, to get better, and you can make an easy connection with them. Parents, though, are entrusting their precious child to you, and they may not fully understand what's going on. They're the ones who need the most guidance, reassurance and support."

HALEY HOOG, R.N.

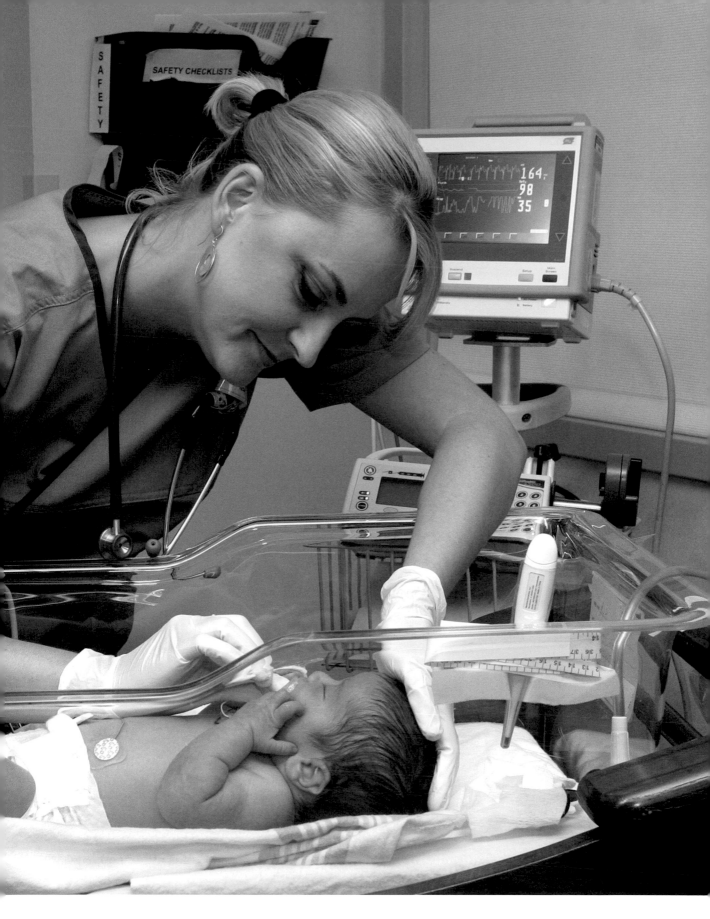

CARING

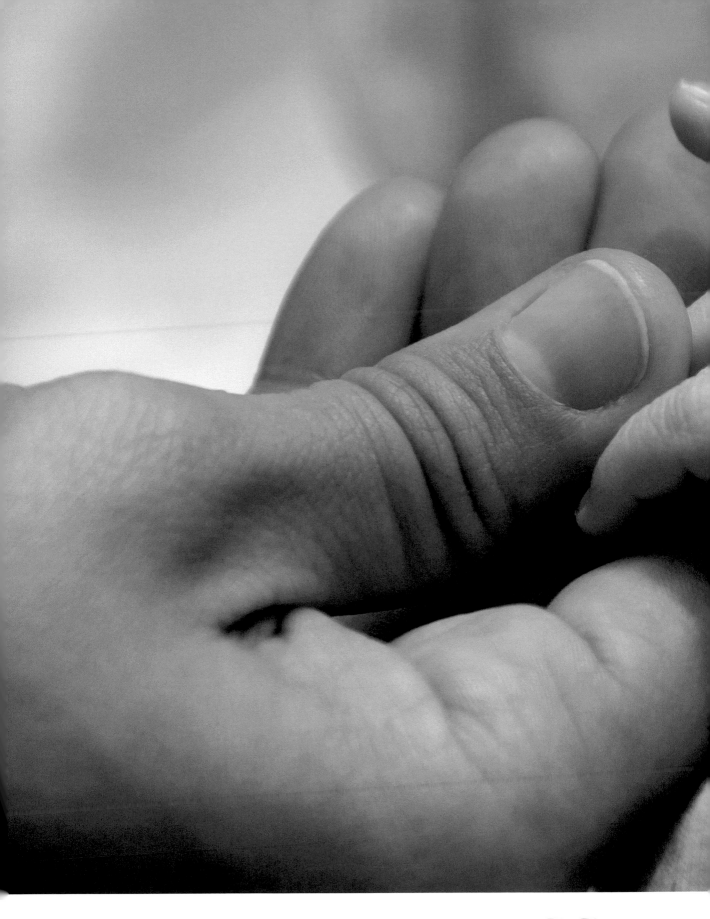

GENTLENESS

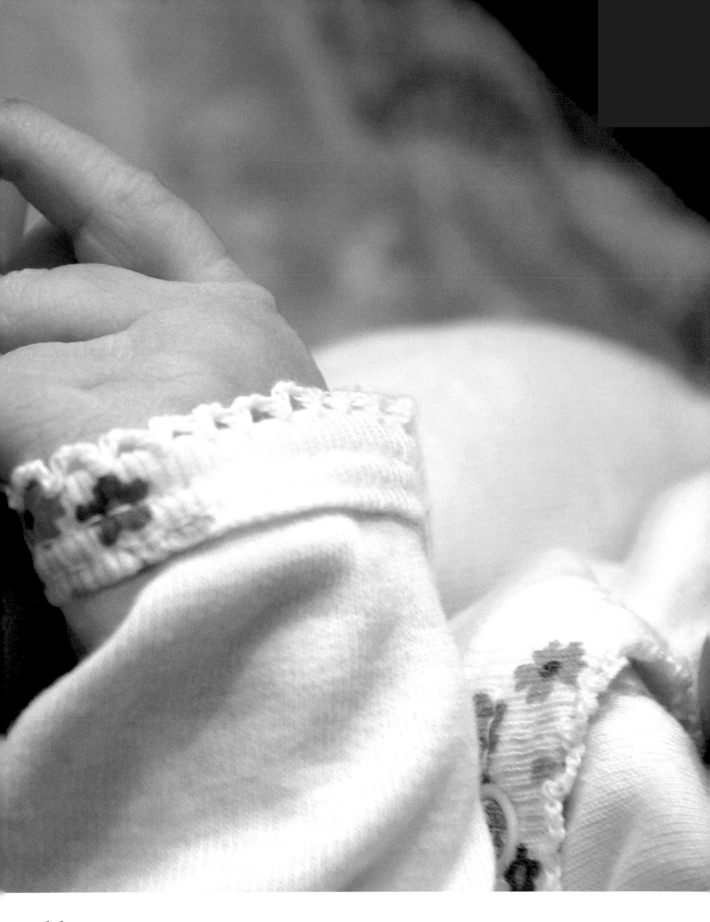

" *Medicine works, but there are so many other aspects of care that affect the well-being of the patient. Just a simple touch or hug can go a long way to provide comfort and ease anxiety.* "

RAY BARNETT, R.N.

changing in appearance, nature or character…

TRANSFORMATIVE

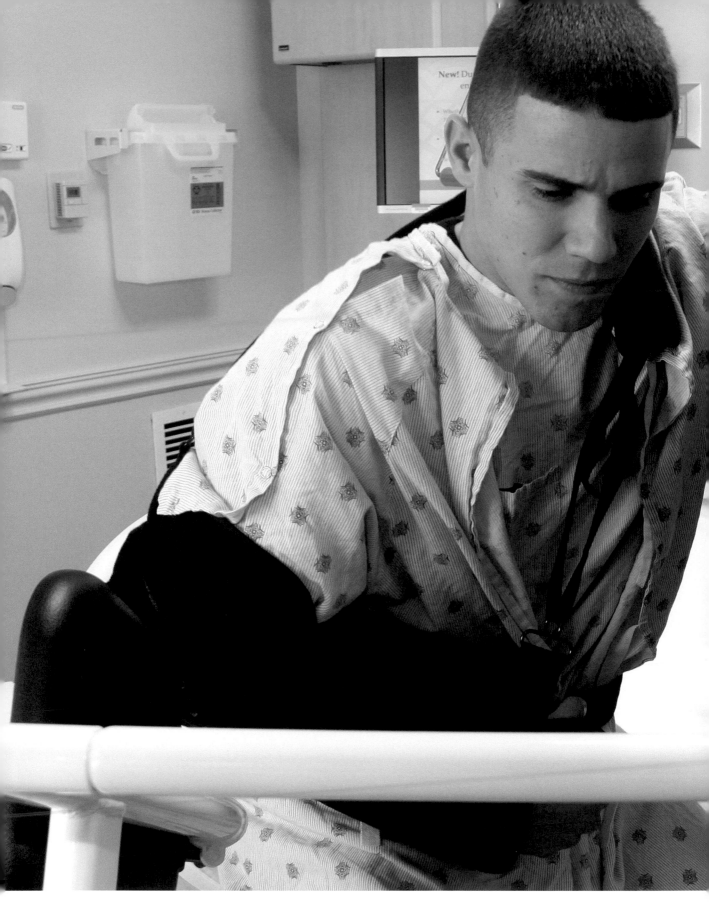

ENDURANCE

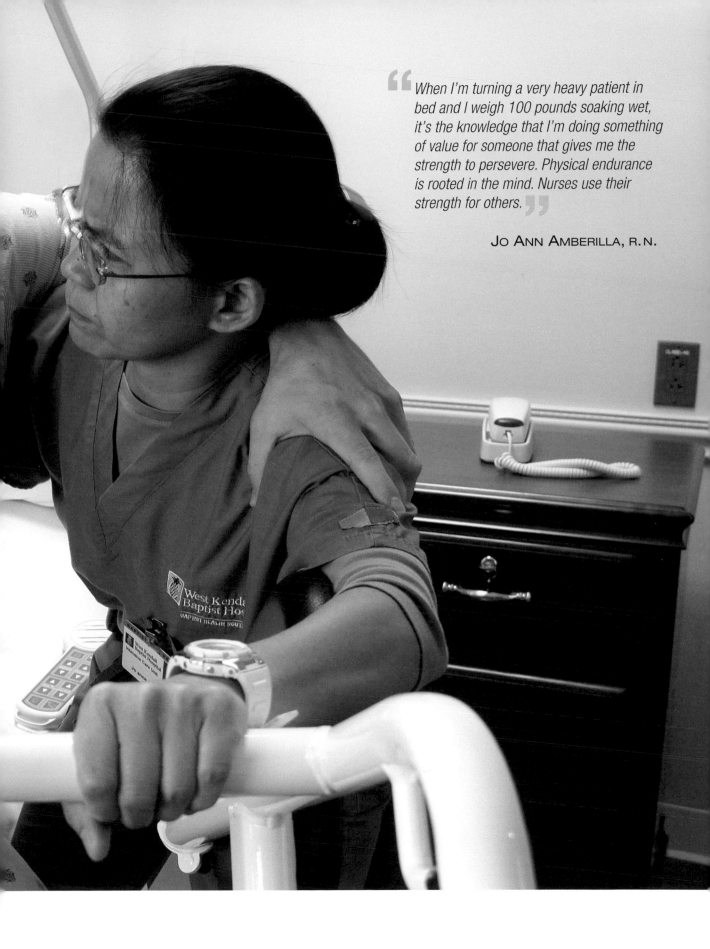

> *When I'm turning a very heavy patient in bed and I weigh 100 pounds soaking wet, it's the knowledge that I'm doing something of value for someone that gives me the strength to persevere. Physical endurance is rooted in the mind. Nurses use their strength for others.*

JO ANN AMBERILLA, R.N.

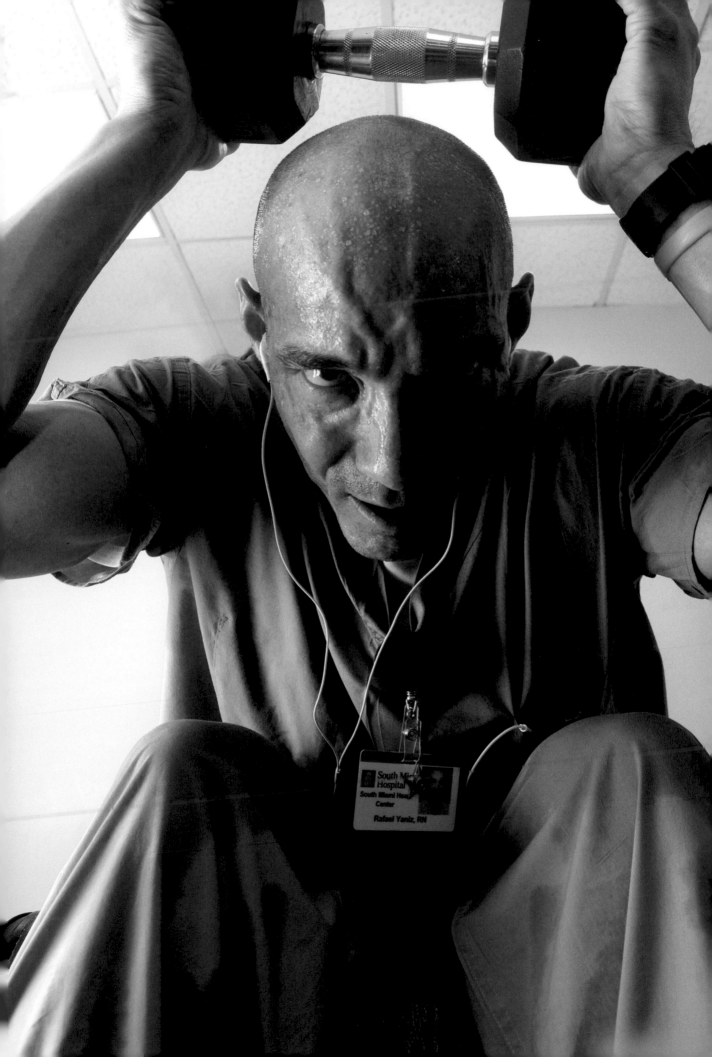

"When you're wheeling equipment and walking those halls every day, it's important to have enough energy and endurance to get through a 12-hour shift. Exercise helps keep your mind focused and fresh. I get up early and exercise before my brain can talk me out of it."

DEBRA CHANEY, R.N.

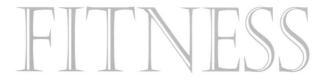

FITNESS

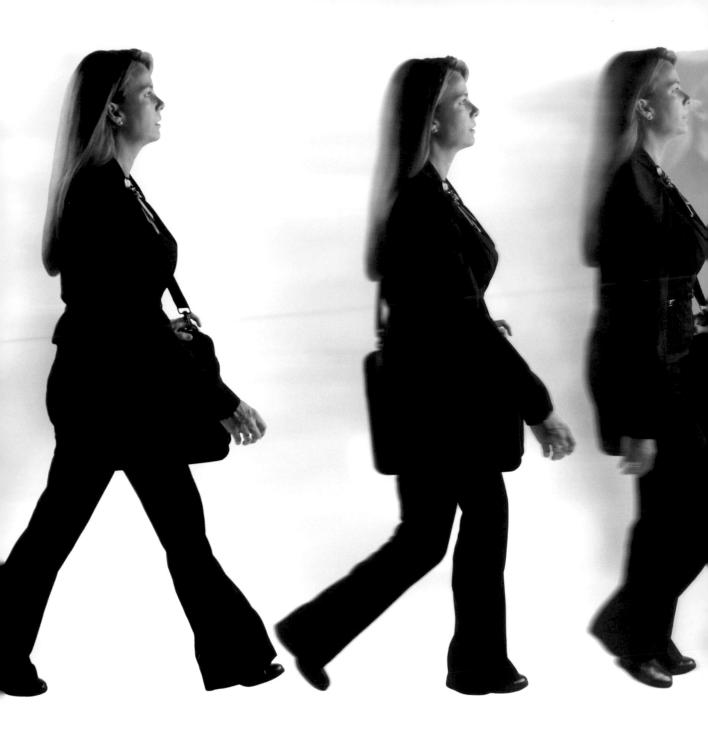

"I'm often approached by young people who want to know if nursing could be a good career for them. I tell them, no matter what your interests are, there's a place for you in nursing. So many doors open as one advances in a nursing career. Whether you want to work with the elderly or help deliver babies, there's a place. Whether you want to sit at a desk or be in the emergency room action, there's a place.

There's the broad range of skills that a nurse must exhibit when with the patient, then there's the whole other world of responsibilities that occur away from the bedside. You have to adjust to so many outside influences. This profession is the definition of versatility."

TINA JONES, R.N.

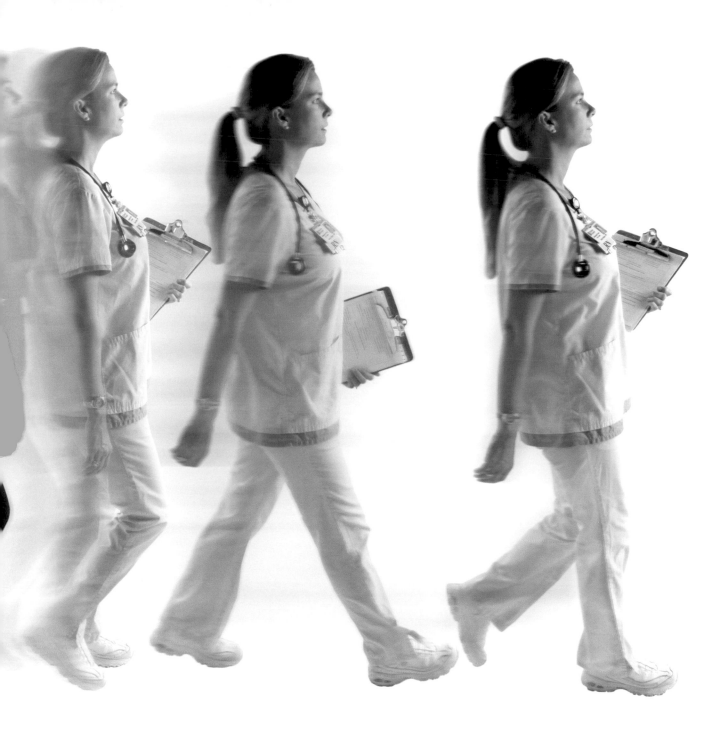

VERSATILITY

"Nursing is absolutely the best career in terms of helping you find yourself and being able to use all of yourself — your intellectual, emotional, physical and spiritual selves — in your work. You keep searching for balance in all of these areas as you grow and situations change."

KATHRYN BISHOPRIC, R.N.

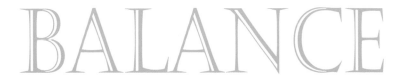

BALANCE

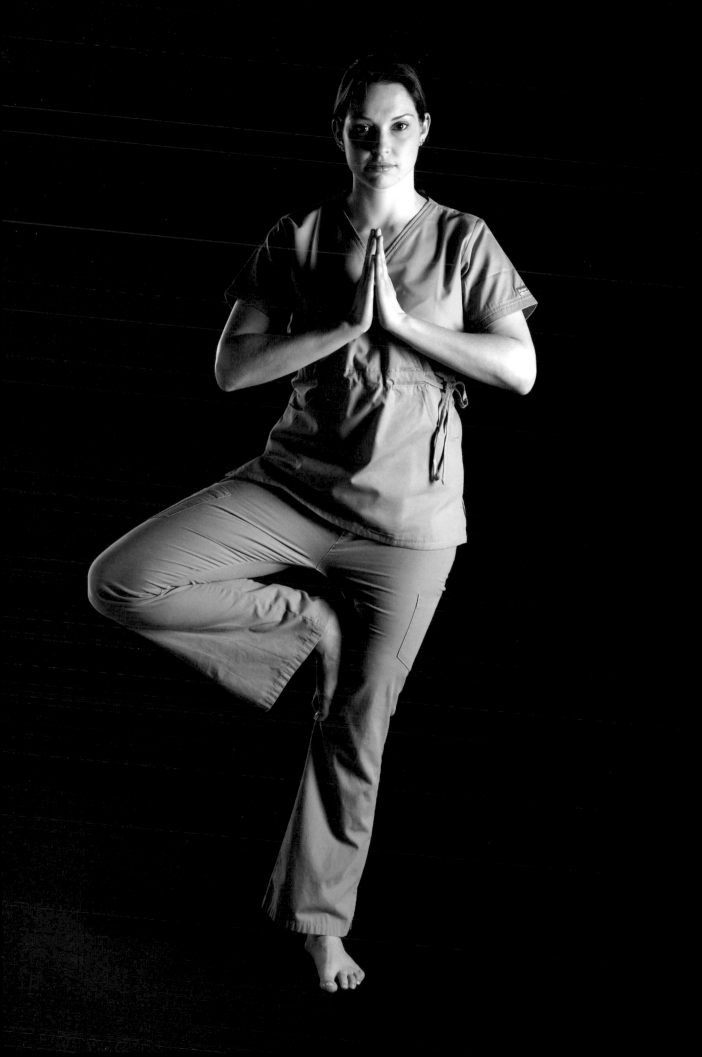

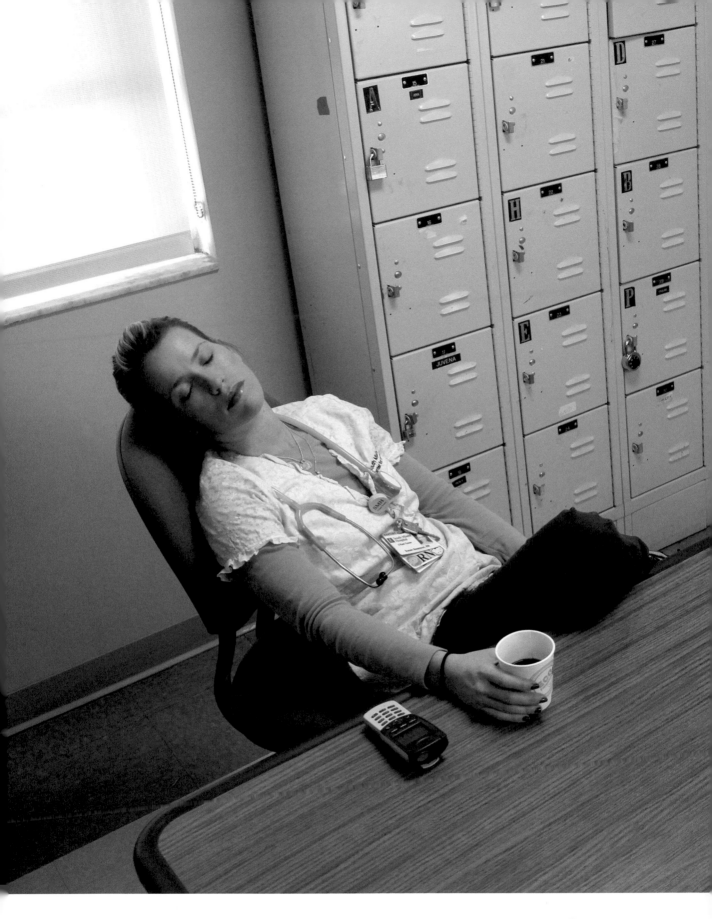

REJUVENATION

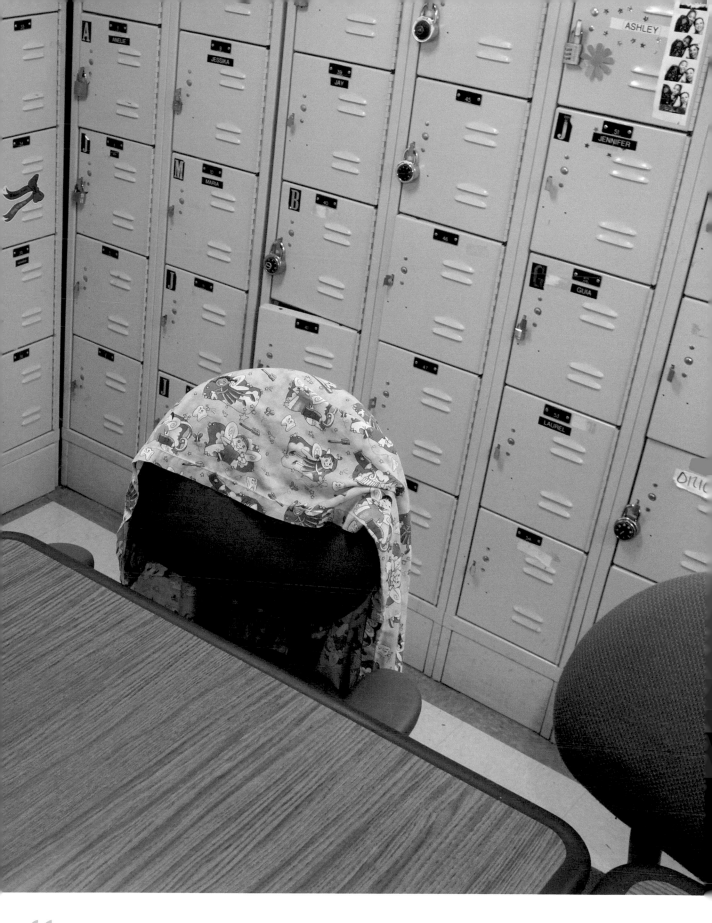

Both my wife and I are nurses. Some days we come home laughing, some days crying and some days so exhausted we can barely speak. We work hard to find those moments when we can actually unplug. When I open my front door and my two little boys are fighting to jump on Daddy, it makes everything worth it.

CARLOS DELGADO, R.N.

*cherishing a
desire with
anticipation...*

HOPEFUL

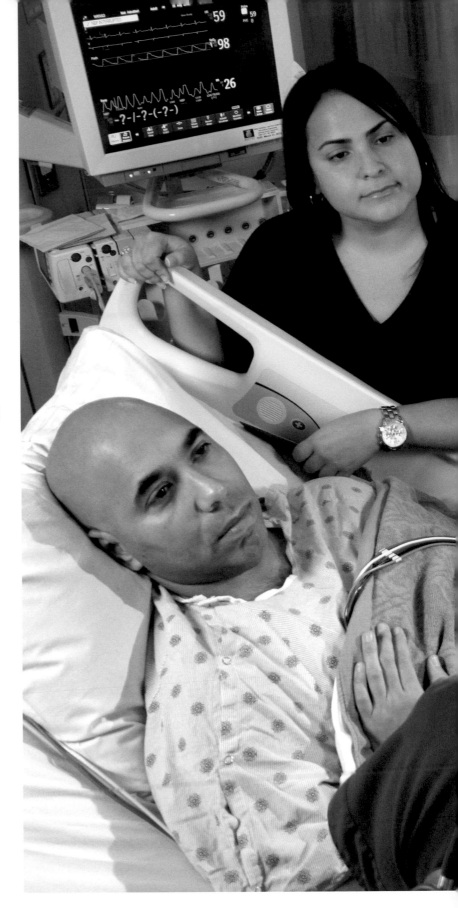

We certainly know from surveys that nursing is seen as the most trusted profession. People show a certain degree of reverence toward our profession by putting themselves in our hands when they are their most vulnerable. Our interaction with patients is like being 'intimate strangers.' We've never met, but inside of half an hour, we know things about a patient that most people on the planet never will know.

CONNIE BARDEN, R.N.

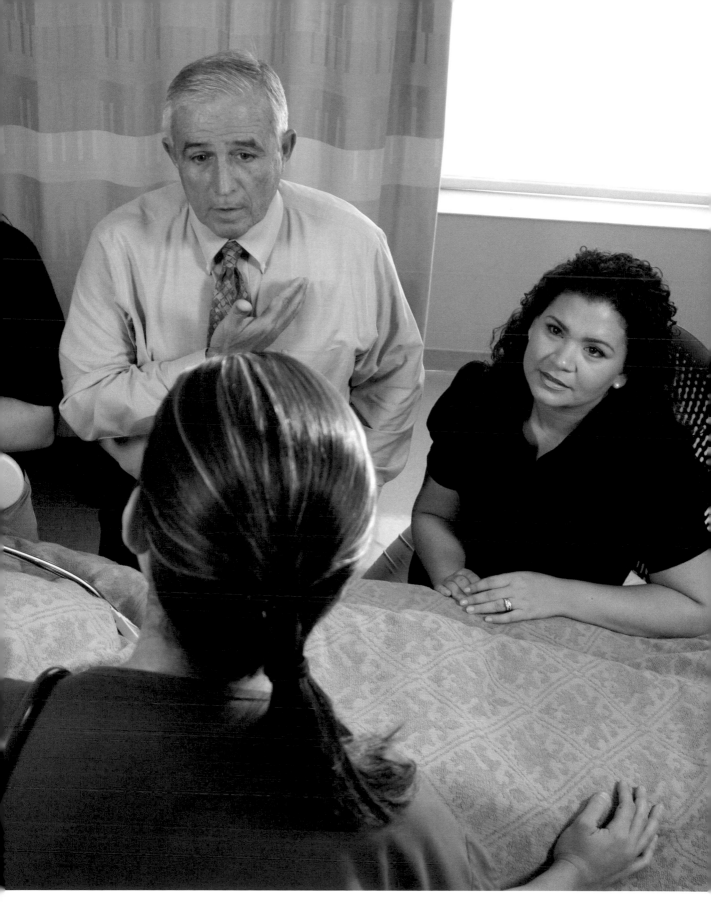

REVERENCE

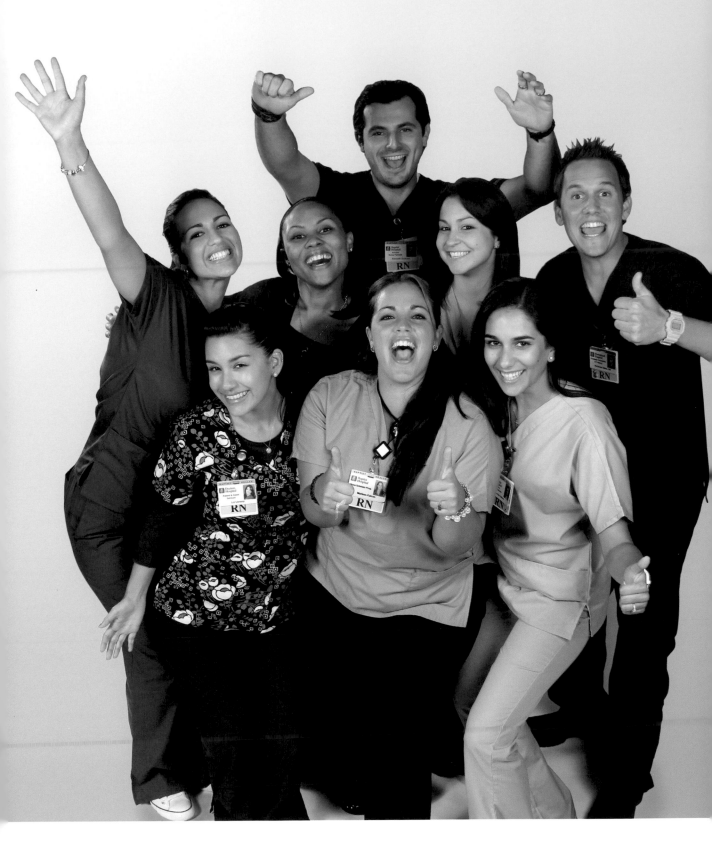

JOY

"*In nursing, every day is different. I continually learn new things about life, and about myself and other people. As an OR nurse, I am often the first face a patient sees after waking up from surgery. It gives me great joy to be there to provide comfort and care.***"**

JESSICA KORNBLATH, R.N.

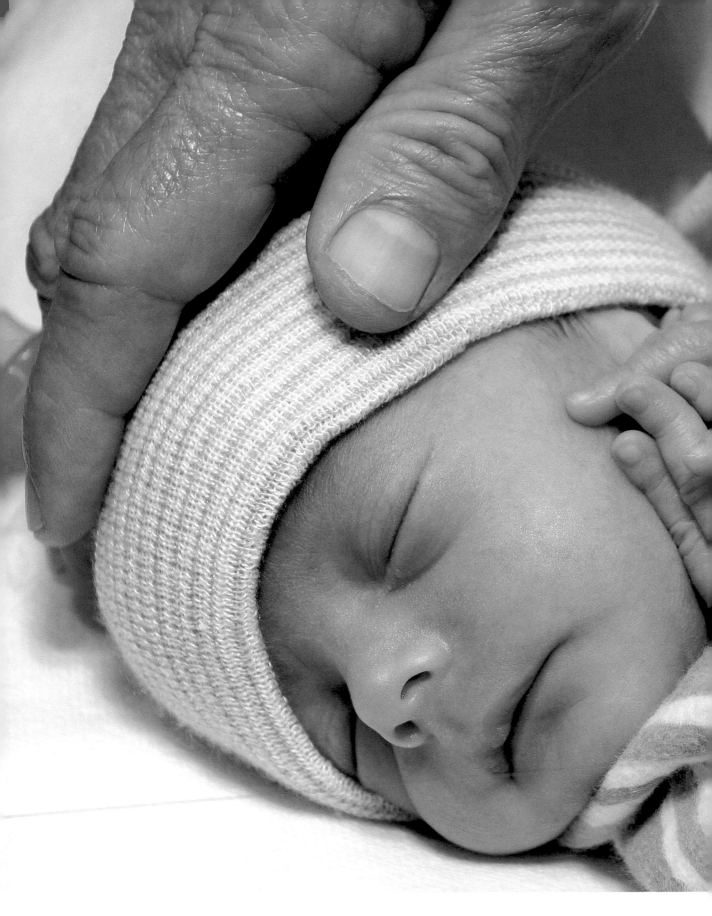

TENDERNESS

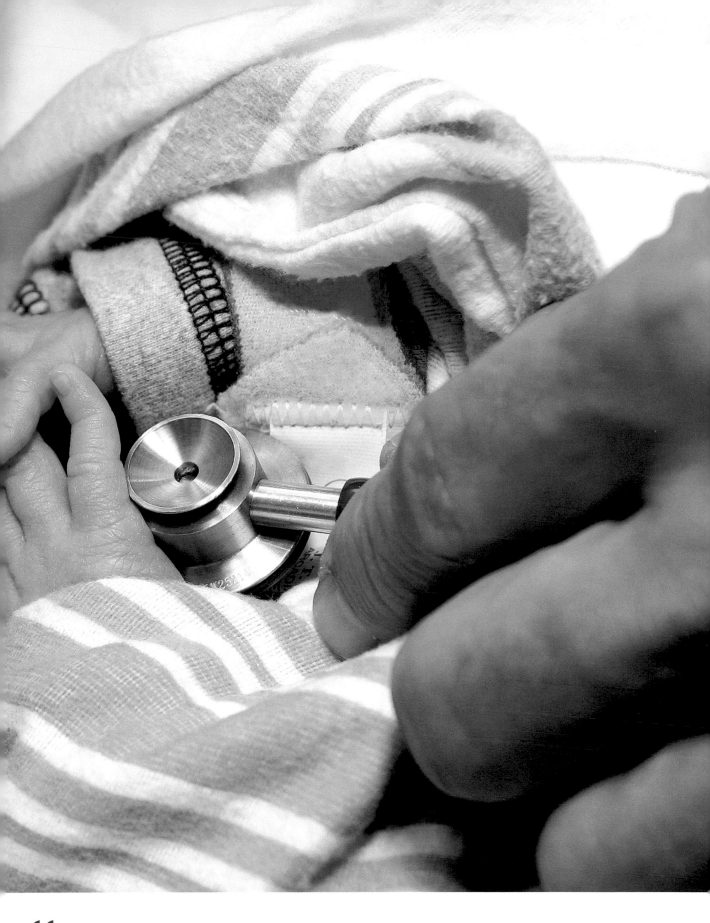

“About 20 years ago, when I was a housewife in Jamaica, my young son was critically injured and hospital-ized for about a week. During that time I never left his bedside. Seeing the tenderness and care the nurses showed my son day after day sparked my desire to seek a career as a nurse. I wanted to be able to do for someone else what those nurses had done for my family.”

ANN MULLINGS, R.N.

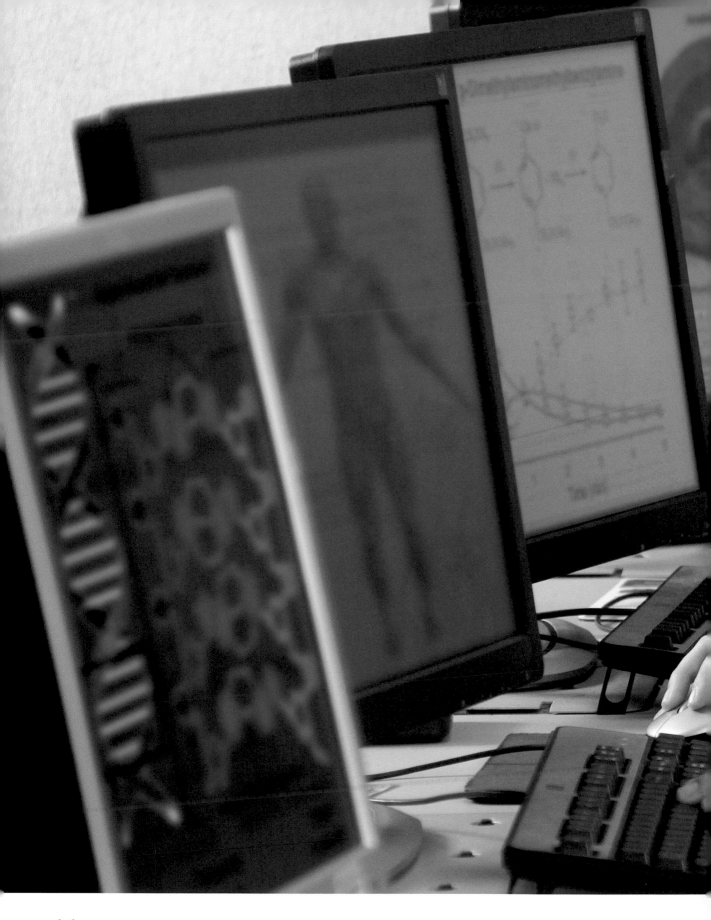

"_Research is part of every nurse's daily practice; they just may not realize it. It is exciting to see more nurses growing into independent researchers who use critical thinking skills and choose research as an avenue to help answer their questions._**"**

TANYA JUDKINS-COHN, R.N.

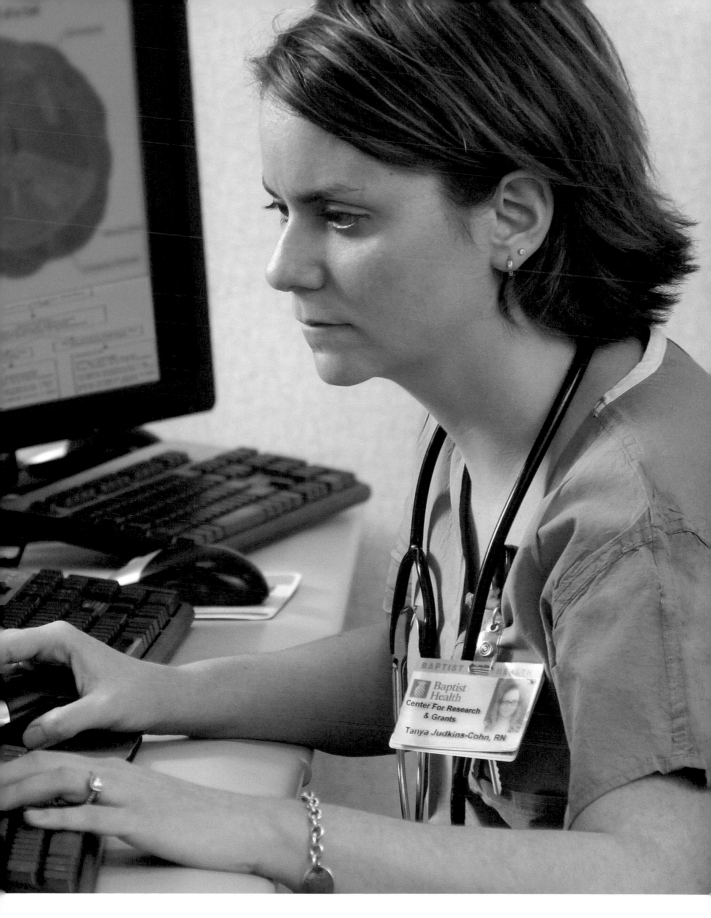

CURIOSITY

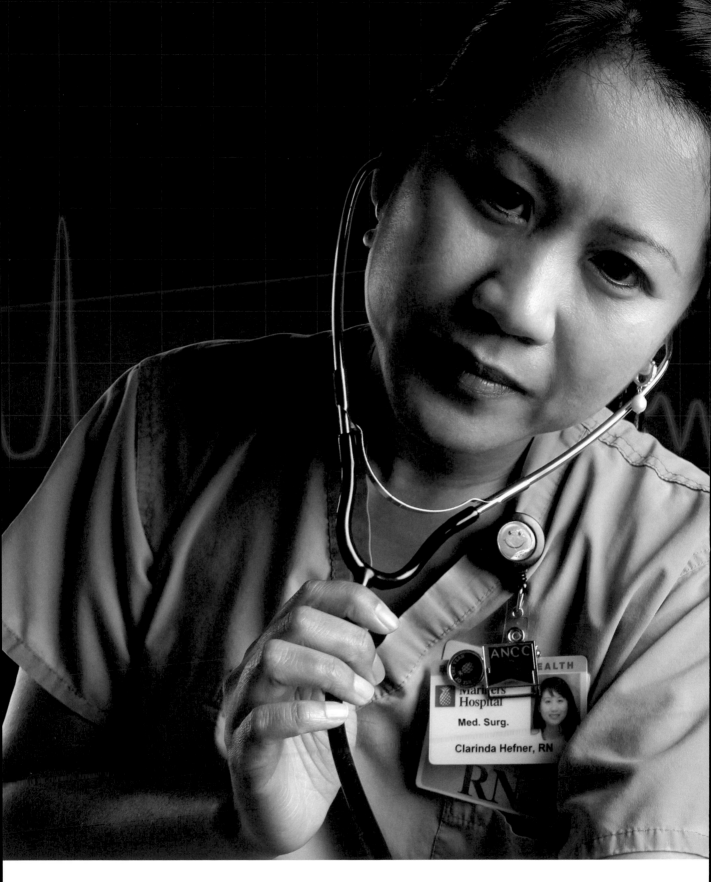

HEARTBEAT

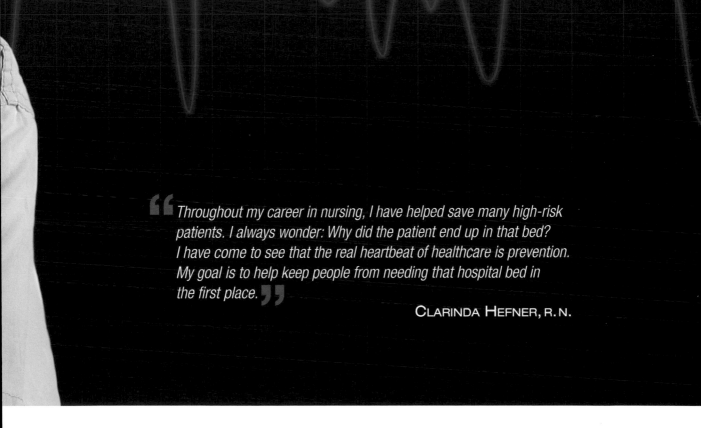

"*Throughout my career in nursing, I have helped save many high-risk patients. I always wonder: Why did the patient end up in that bed? I have come to see that the real heartbeat of healthcare is prevention. My goal is to help keep people from needing that hospital bed in the first place.*"

CLARINDA HEFNER, R.N.

OF HEALTHCARE

99

concerned with the conscious life or the soul...

SPIRITUAL

"Nurses have the ability to celebrate and embrace patients in one moment and console them as they grieve in the next. We meet people during some of the happiest times in their lives as well as some of the most difficult. Nurses care for complete strangers and treat them as friends. It is not just a career but also a way of life."

NATALIE VOGT, R.N.

RADIANCE

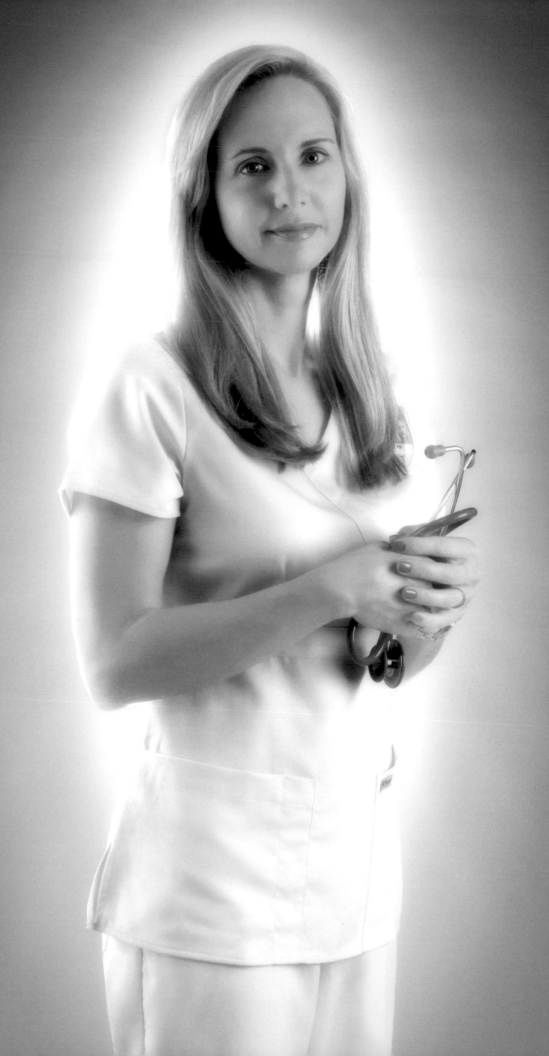

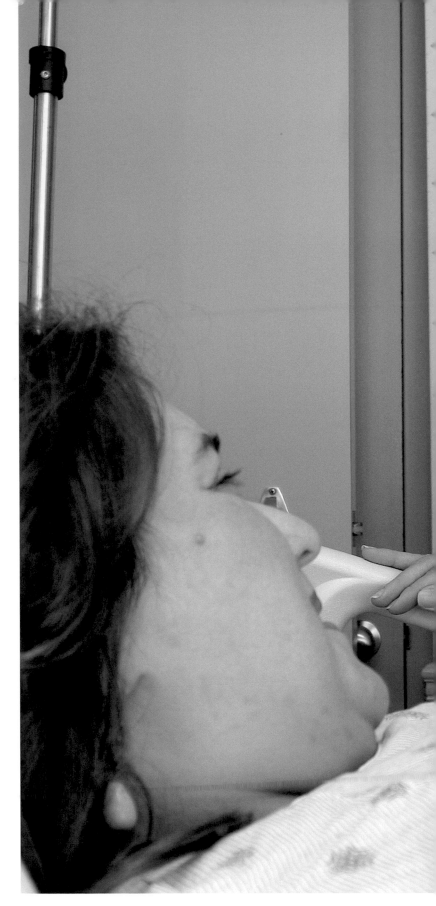

"When you make the commitment to go into nursing, you're committing to help mankind. It's not a glamorous job, and it is not about the paycheck — it's how you feel when you make a difference in someone else's day or life. And that happens every day.

I once stepped into an elevator and a woman said to me, 'I know you. You saved my husband's life.' She described in detail a situation that happened years before, that I didn't even remember. It was a powerful moment for me."

GAIL GORDON, R.N.

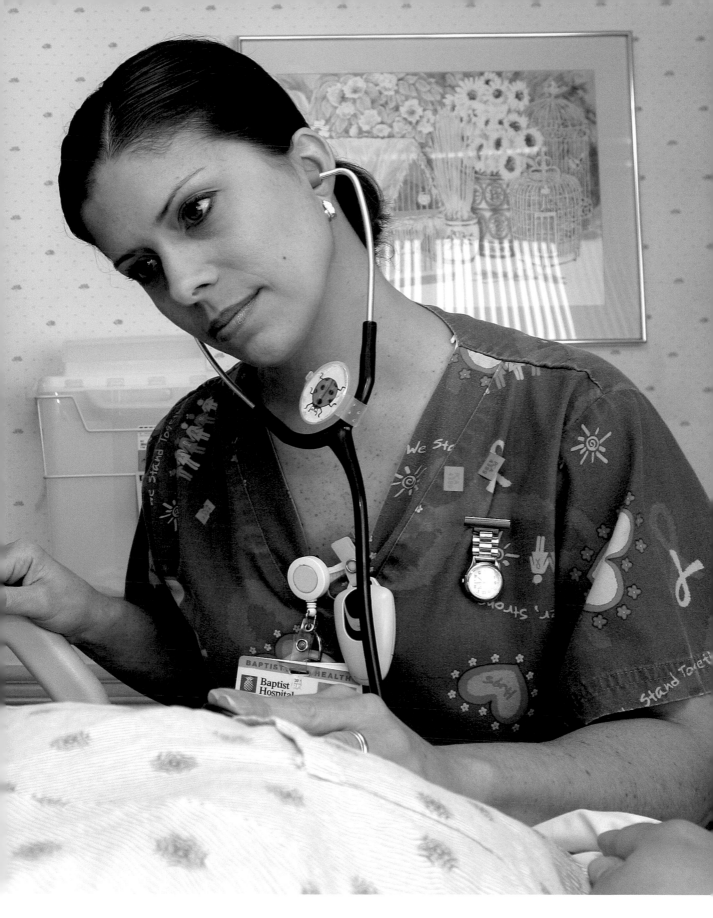

HUMANITY

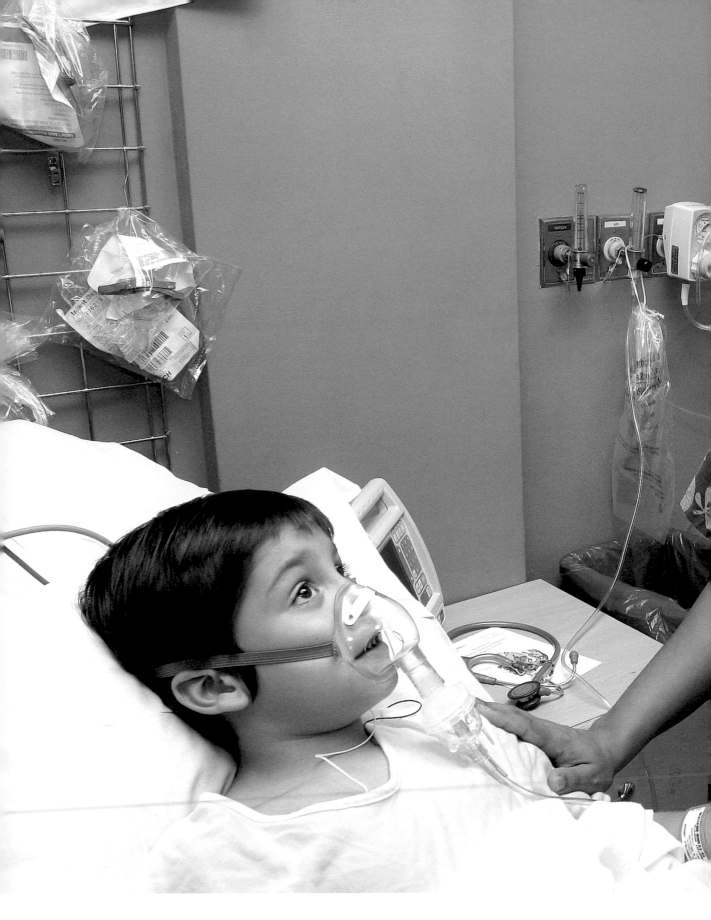

"So many times I've sat with patients who have received bad news. I just hold their hand and say, 'Cry. You are going through something that will happen to all of us. I will sit here as long as you want to cry.'"

LILLIAN GIRAS, R.N.

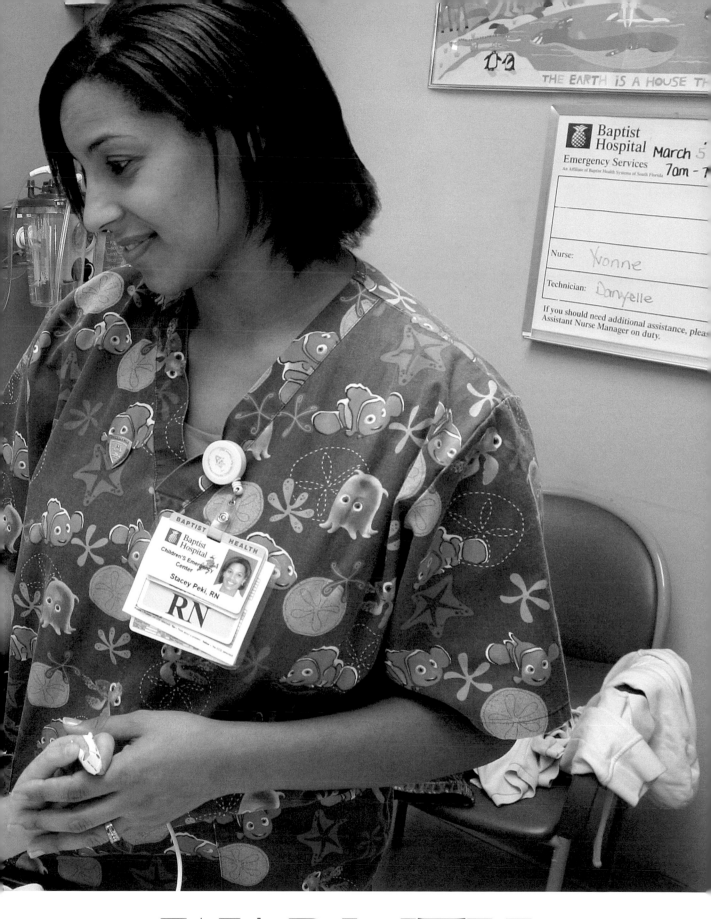

WARMTH

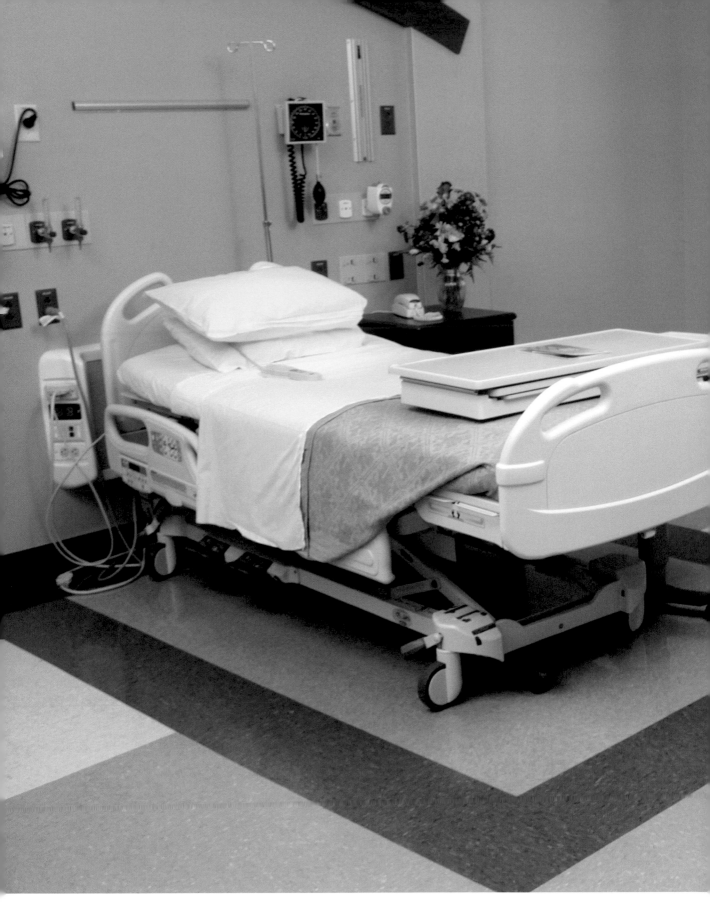

"It's hard to imagine feeling serene in the middle of a busy cardiac unit. There's no downtime to sit and experience such an emotion. However, when you find that calmness within yourself, you can transfer it to a patient who is having a negative experience. It's an innate ability nurses develop without really noticing."

SHENNY CORDERO, R.N.

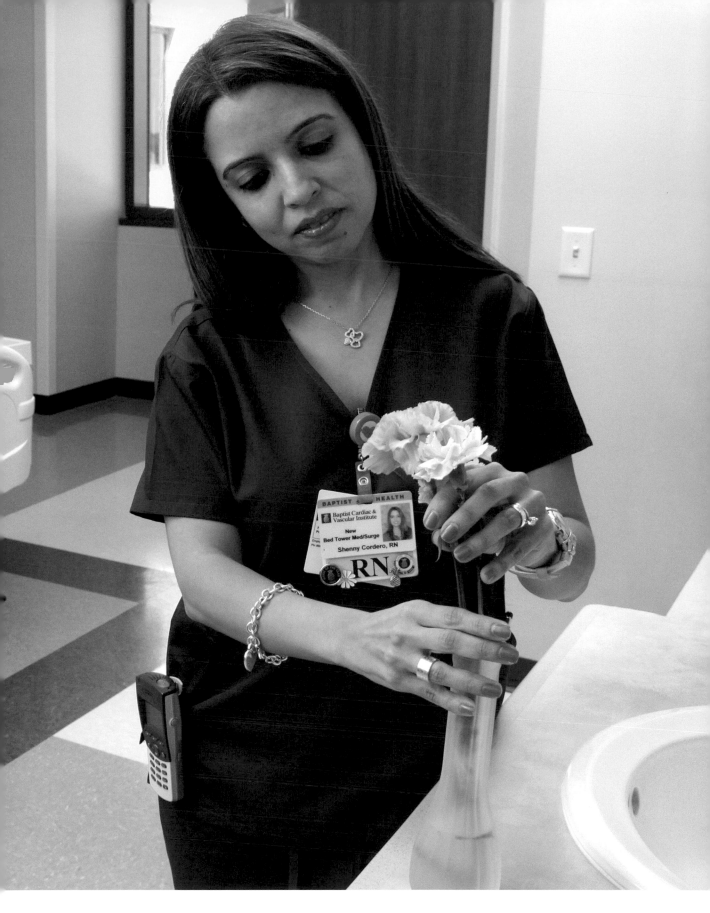

SERENITY

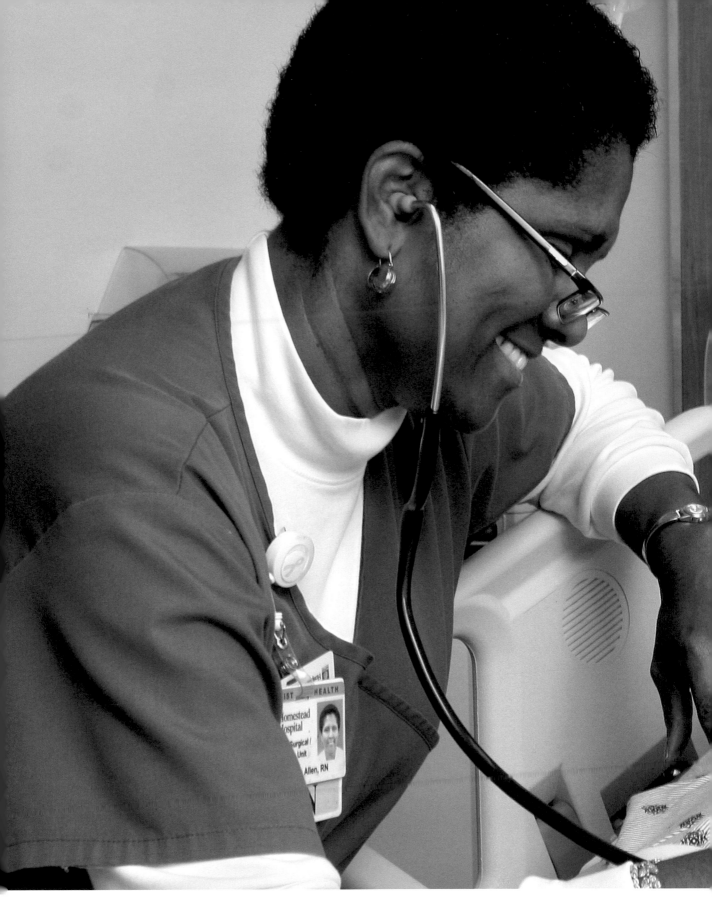

HEALING

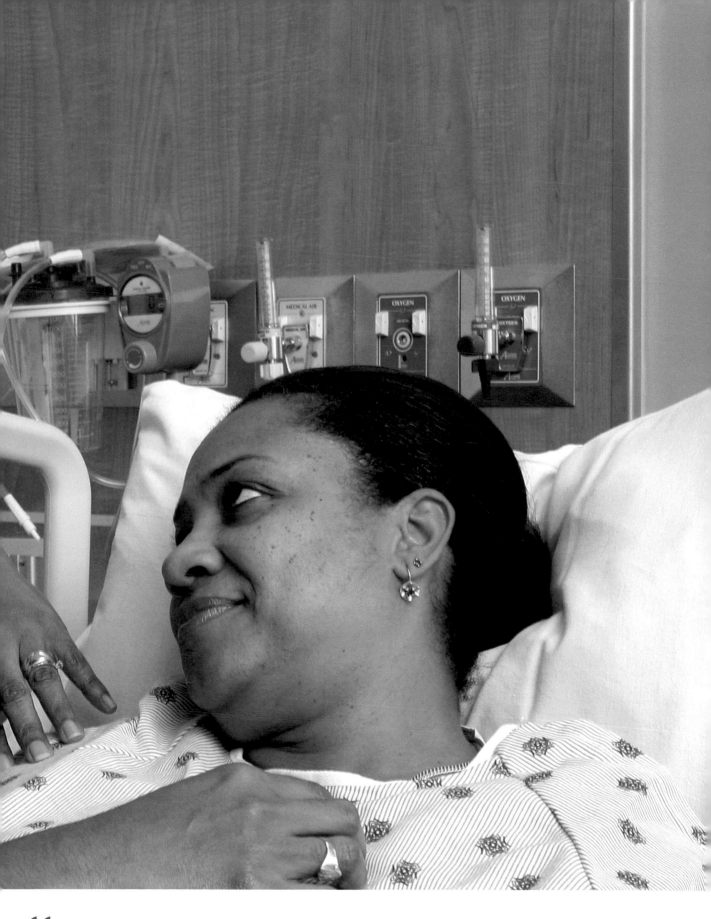

"The nurse's role is to draw out the coping mechanisms of the patient. We need to know how they deal with adversity so we can help them begin to heal. Healing doesn't necessarily mean they are cured. It's more that they know they are doing everything they can to make the best of their life — to let go of anger, disregard the minutiae and appreciate every day they have."

CINDY BOWLING, R.N.

111

recovering readily from adversity, rebounding...

RESILIENT

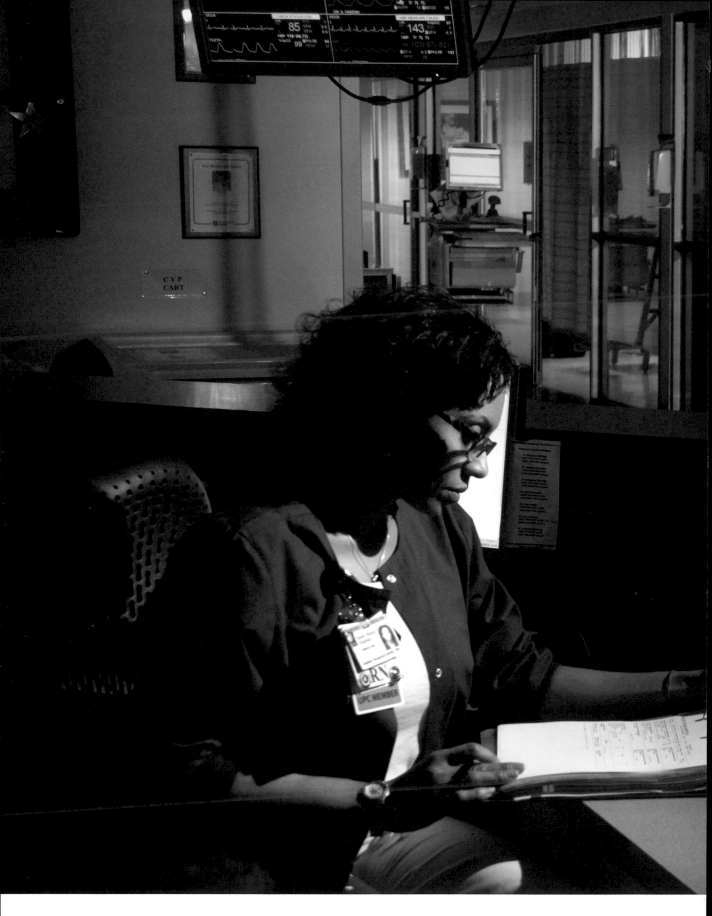

CONSTANCY

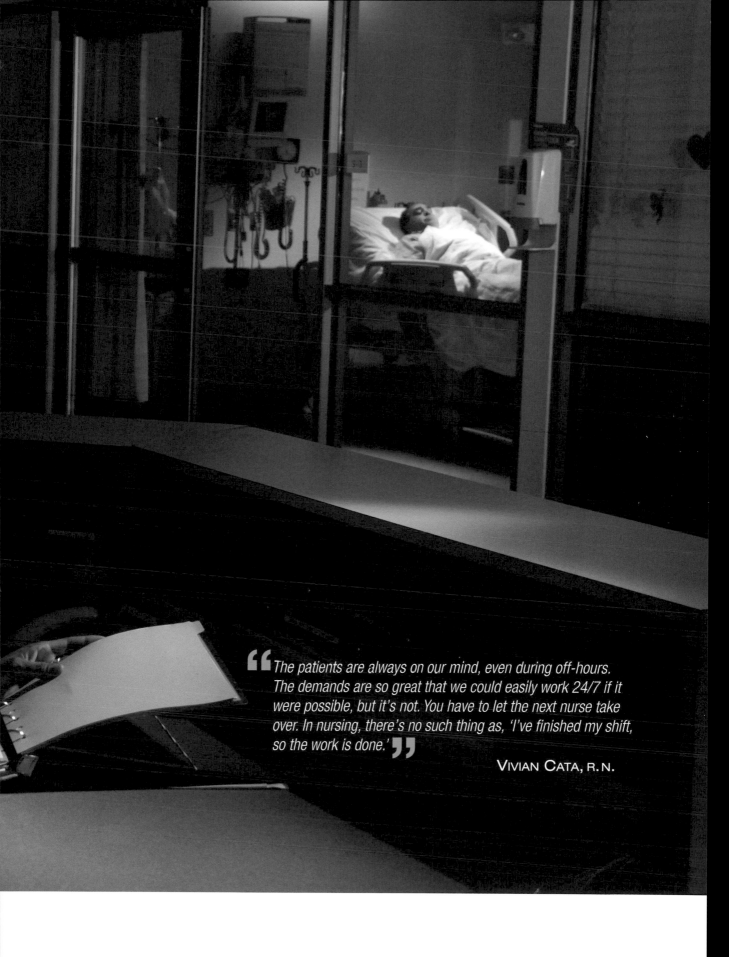

"The patients are always on our mind, even during off-hours. The demands are so great that we could easily work 24/7 if it were possible, but it's not. You have to let the next nurse take over. In nursing, there's no such thing as, 'I've finished my shift, so the work is done.'**"**

VIVIAN CATA, R.N.

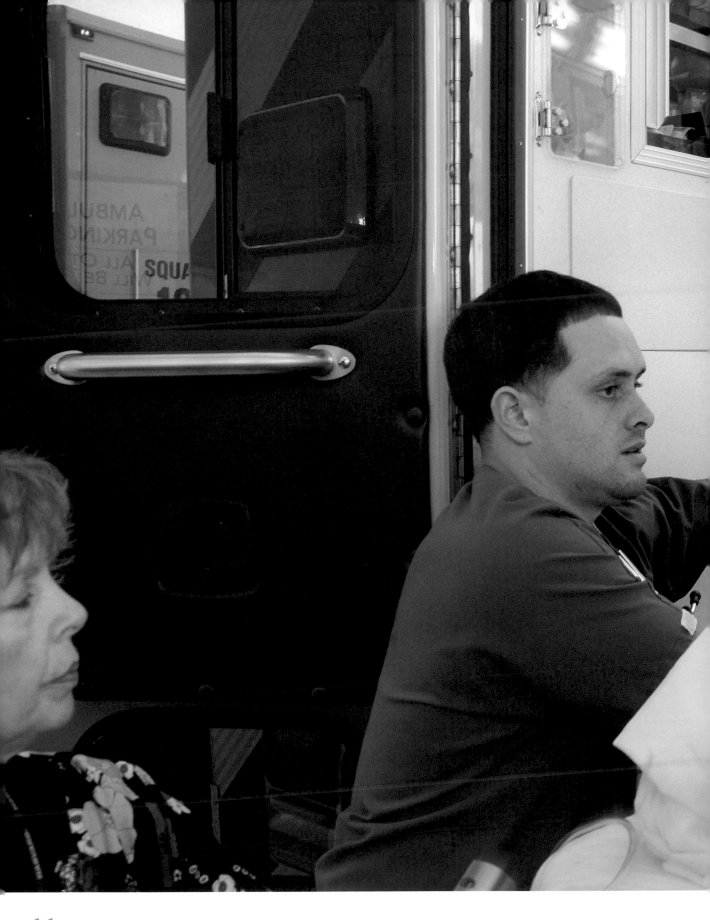

"On the frontline in the emergency department, we have to be prepared for the unexpected. We participate in constant training and education, learning about new treatments and procedures that can help us save lives, so we are ready mentally as well as physically. We know we can handle whatever comes through that door."

JORGE BOLIVAR, R.N.

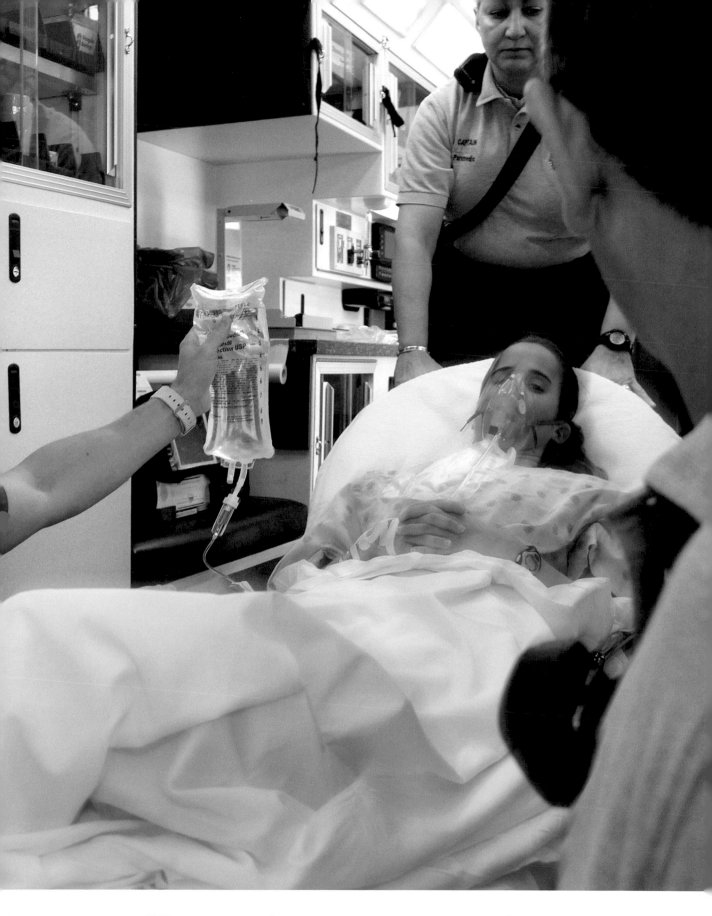

READINESS

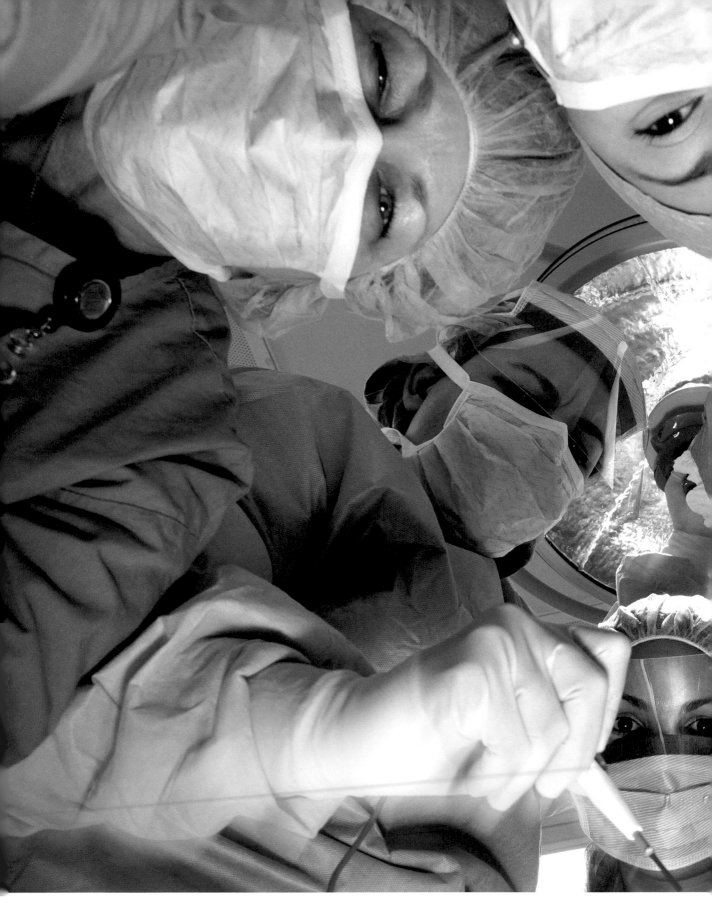

VIGILANCE

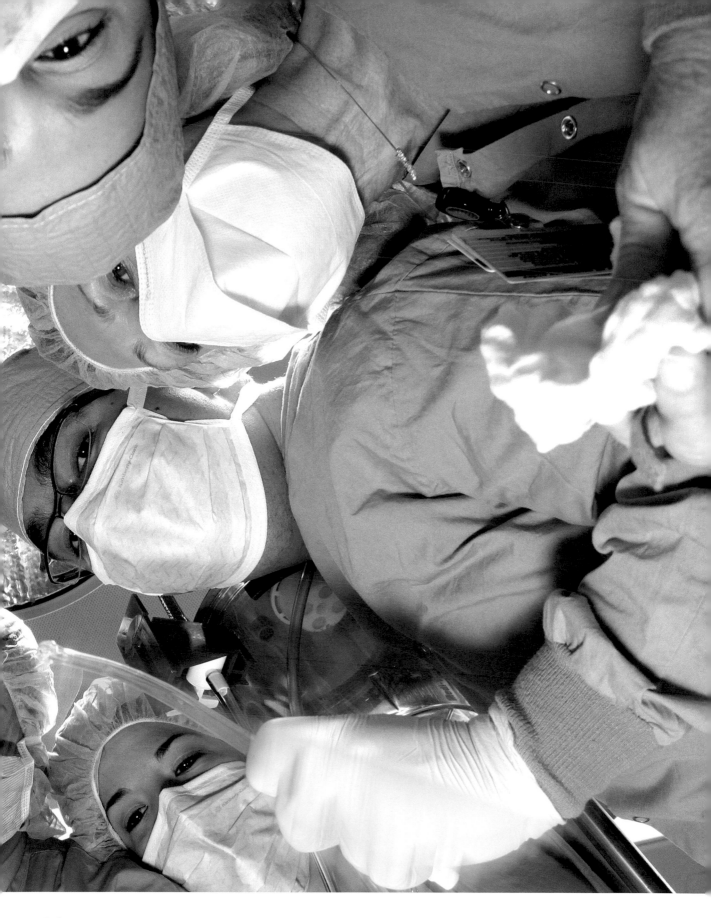

"Some days at our outpatient facility we have 40 patients come in as soon as we open in the morning. The entire staff is engaged and helping each other at all times. You have to realize that one person can't do everything. If you try to handle tough situations on your own, it just doubles the chaos. You have to reach out and accept help."

YENNY CEBALLOS, R.N.

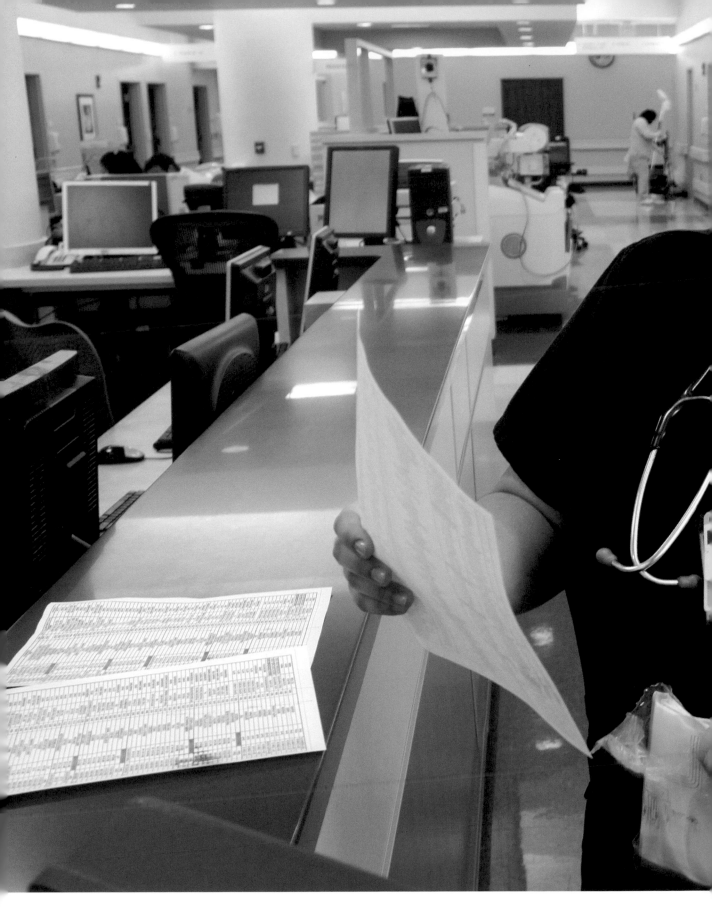

MULTITASKING

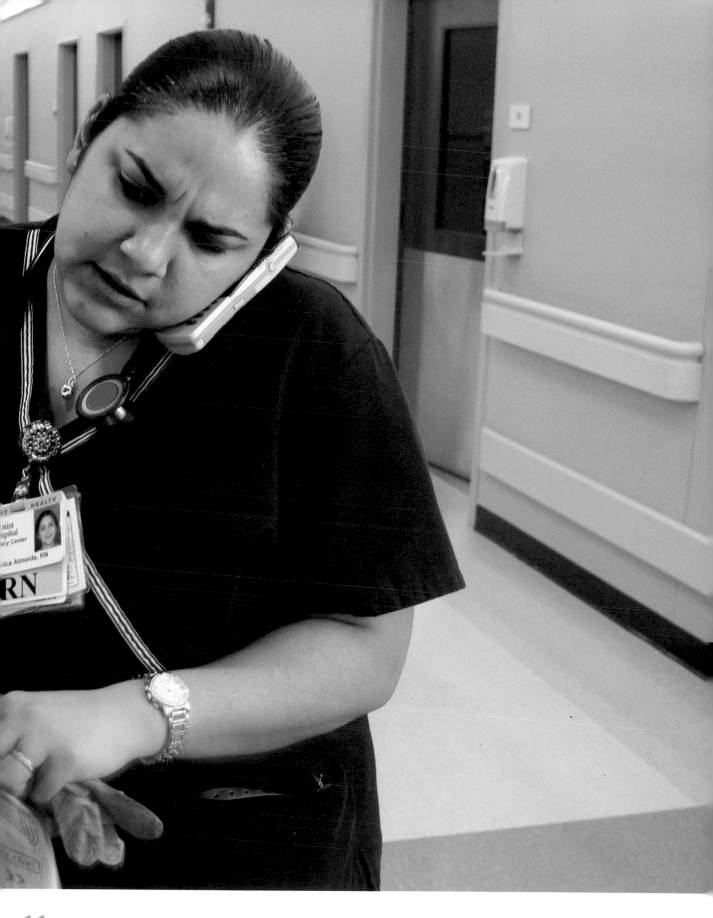

"There are a lot of nurses out there trying to better themselves, continuing their education while dealing with the demands of a family and a full-time job. For me, everything begins at home. If I didn't have the level of support from my family, I wouldn't be able to come to work every day with the right attitude and mindset."

SANDRA JONES, R.N.

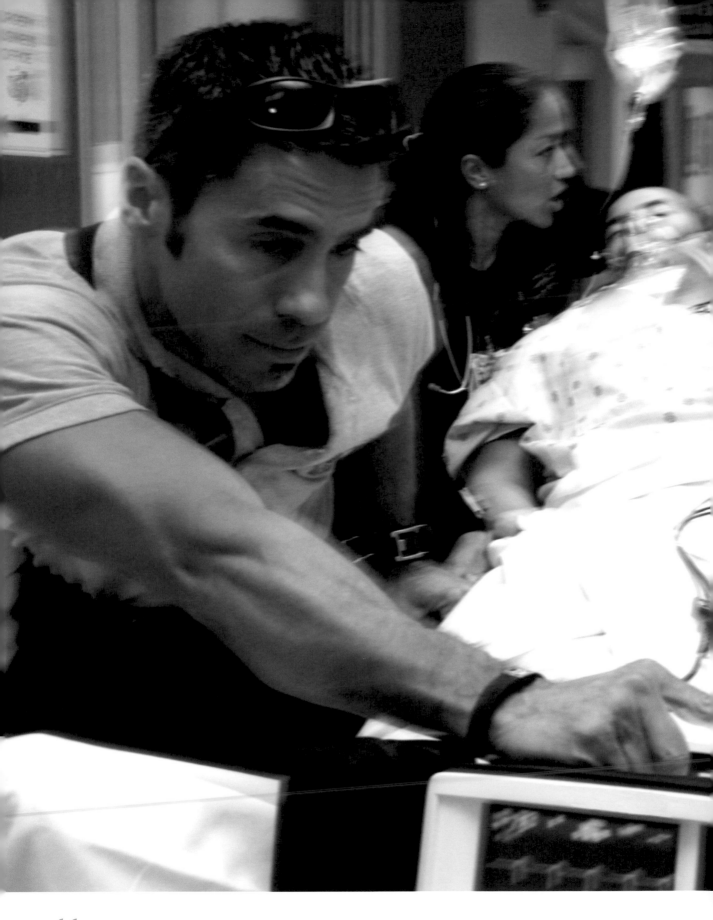

"In the ER, we usually don't have the luxury of time to reflect. We are working together, as a team, at a very fast pace to save someone's life. It feels great when it pays off. You have a lot of those moments where you think, 'Wow, look what I've done.' You can turn someone's life around in seconds."

SILVIA CLARK, R.N.

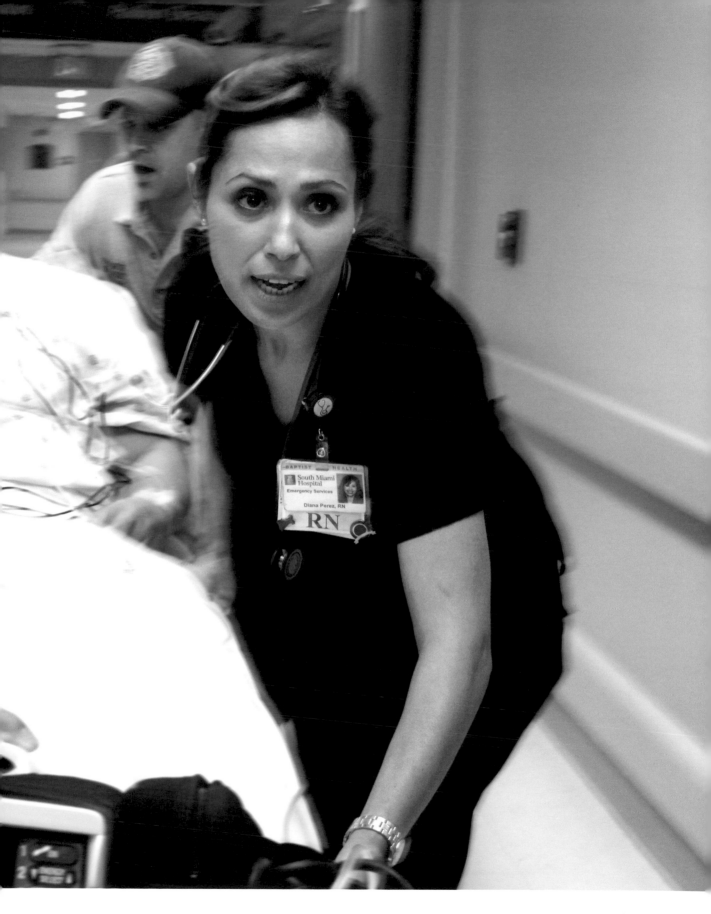

URGENCY

*presenting
a clear or
unmistakable
impression...*

DISTINCTIVE

" *As a new nurse, I have a job that has already given me so many one-of-a-kind experiences. One night, I sat and talked with a very sick patient who shared his life story with me. He passed away later that night. I felt such a sense of gratitude that God had allowed me to share that moment with a stranger.* **"**

JENNIFER LIMA, R.N.

UNIQUENESS

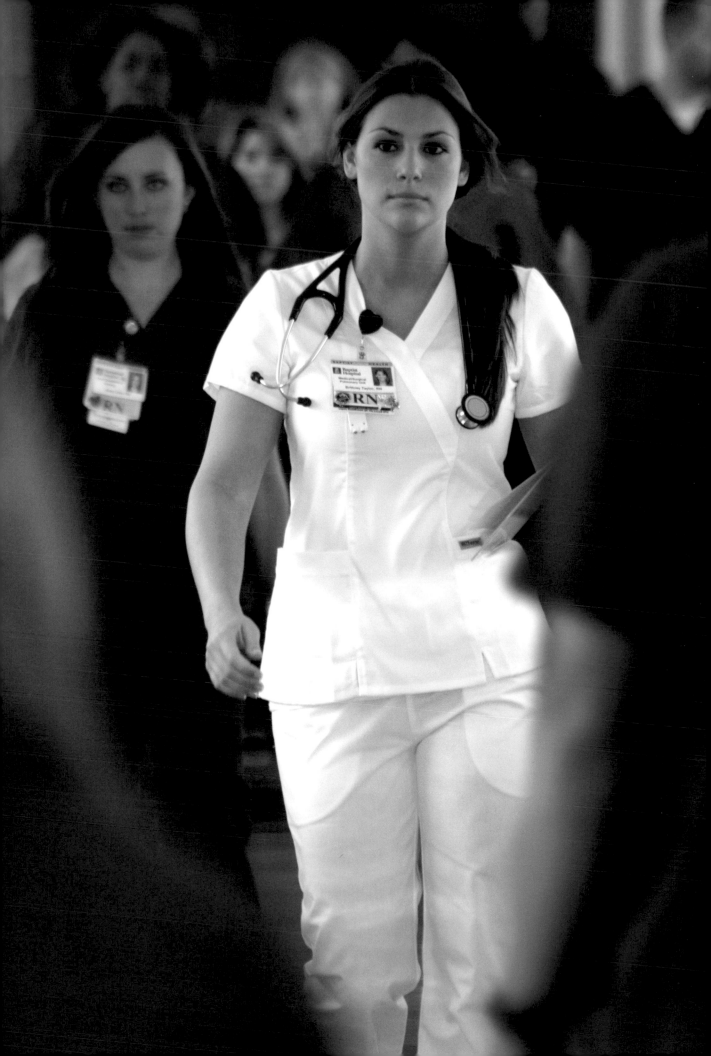

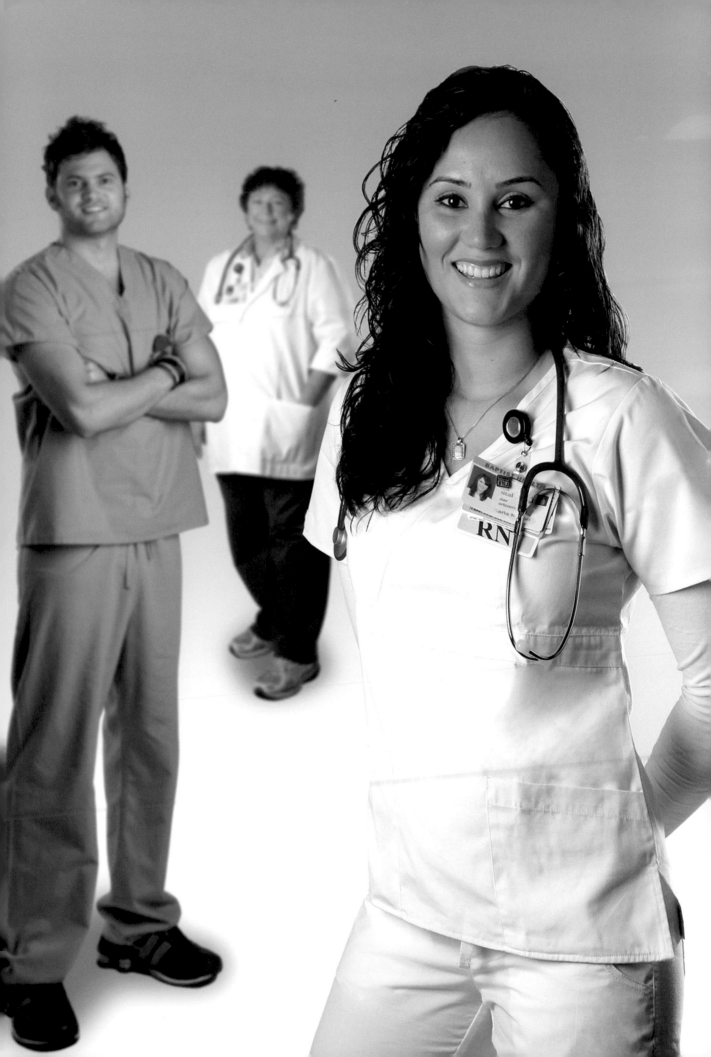

"I remember well the nurse who took the time to train me when I was just beginning my career. She showed me how to organize my shift, to do a clear and concise patient assessment and to plan and anticipate events. She taught me critical thinking. She shared a legacy with me that I value to this day.

In turn, I hope young nurses will remember me as someone who cared, who was committed to their growth as nurses and was an advocate for both patients and our profession."

CHERYL COTTRELL, R.N.

CONTINUITY

"Patients come in every color, creed, culture, age group, income, you name it — but those things really don't matter. We advocate for every patient, as we are all human beings and we want to live peacefully and leave this world as free of pain as we can."

NAYIVE HERNANDEZ, R.N.

DIVERSITY

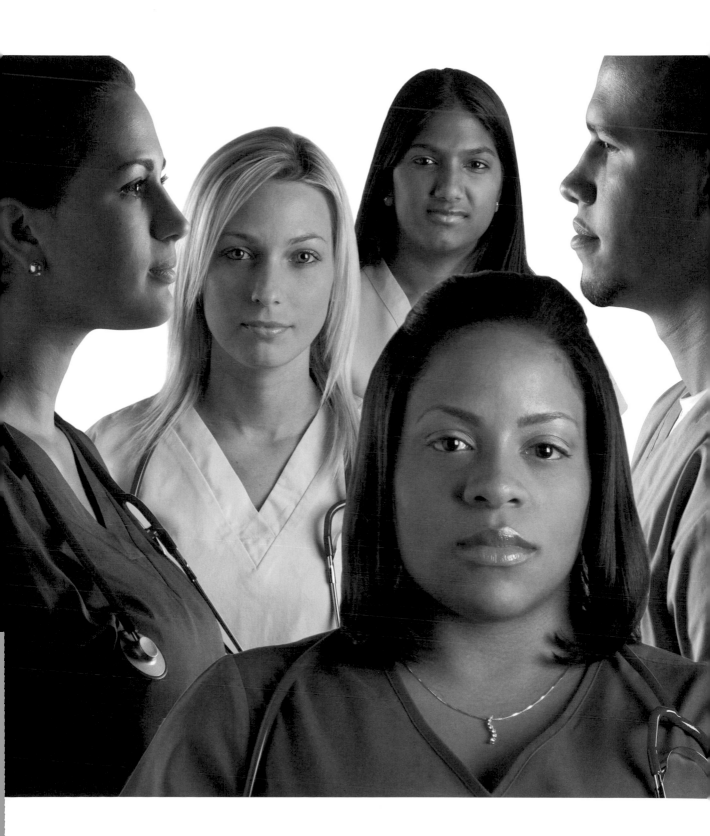

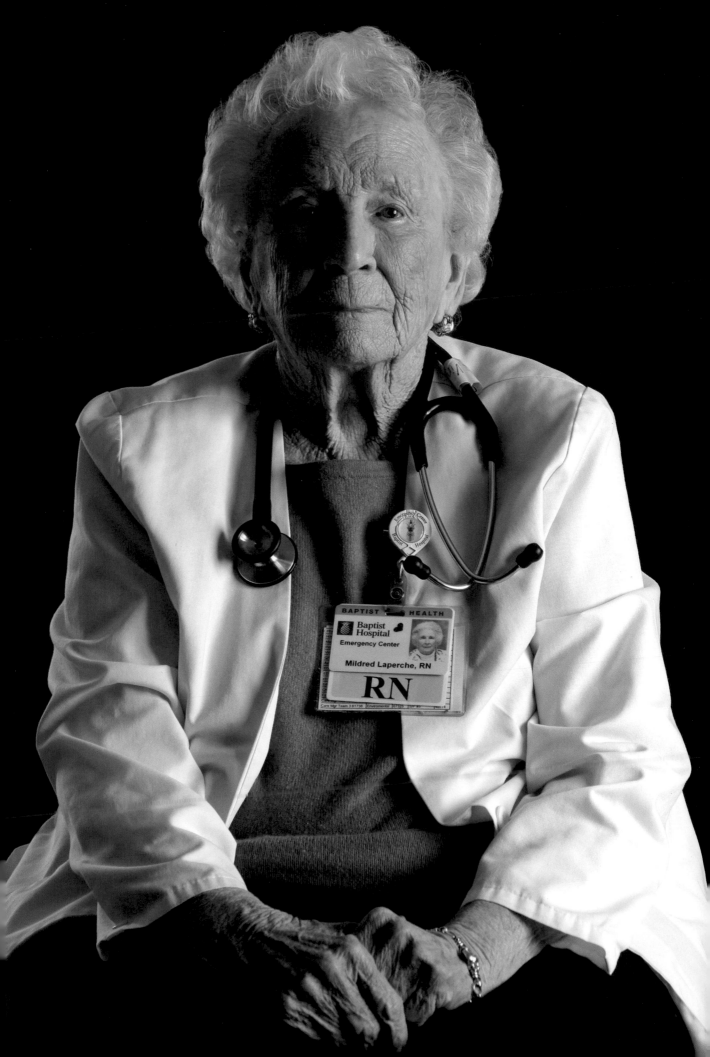

"Nurses who have reached professional maturity have a level of comfort within themselves that they will make sound decisions, yet are still humble enough to ask questions, listen carefully and learn from their mistakes.

I've been a nurse for 40 years, and even now there's not a single day I don't learn something new. With experience comes the ability to think critically — to process new information in order to achieve the best outcomes, and to evaluate the qualities of your team members so you take advantage of everyone's assets."

KATHY SPARGER, R.N.

EXPERIENCE

The healthcare industry and the nursing profession are changing rapidly. In the future, nurses will probably be asked to do more with less and to work in new and unfamiliar environments. We will see an increasing degree of specialization driven by advances in technology.

One aspect of nursing that will not change is our devotion to service. Caring and compassion will remain central to the work we do. The challenge will be to take advantage of the technology while using it with a caring heart.

BECKY MONTESINO, R.N.

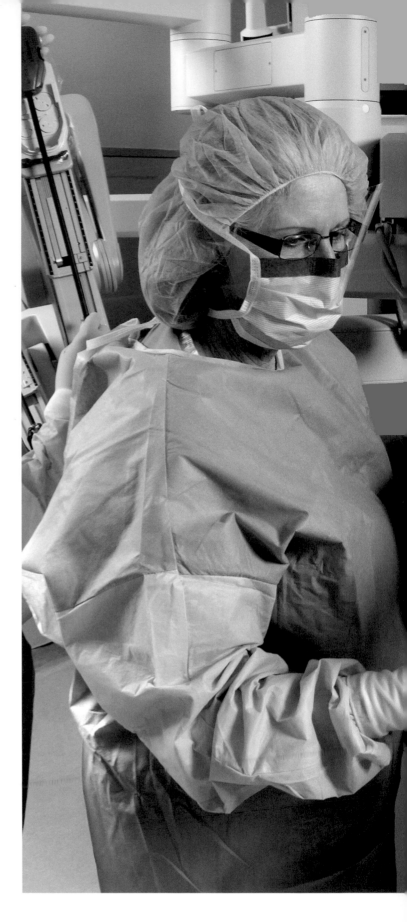

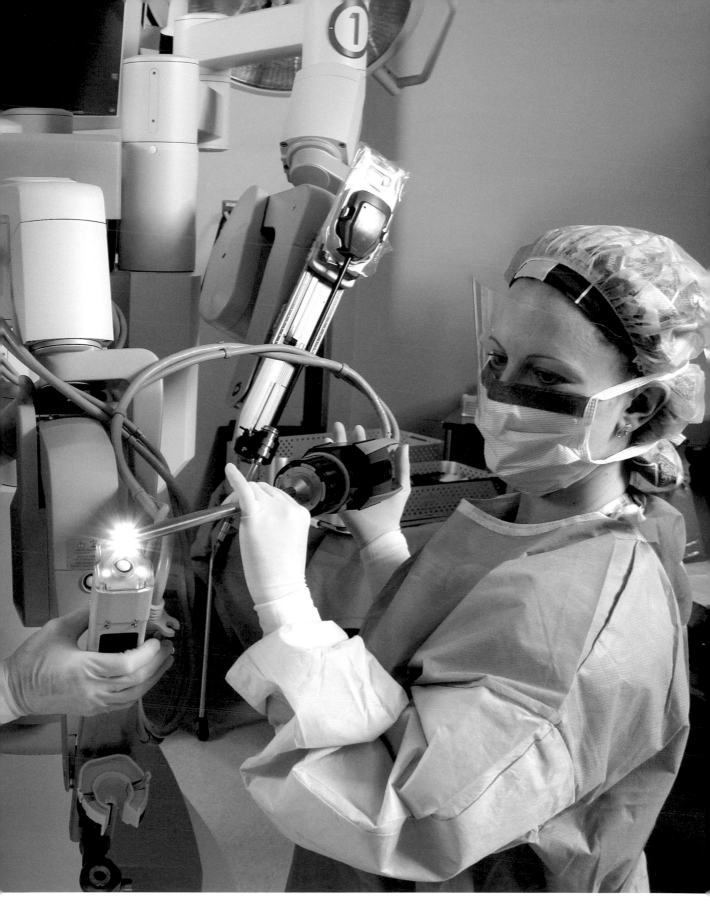

FORESIGHT

PHOTO INDEX

This project would not have been possible without the enthusiastic cooperation of many friends and colleagues throughout Baptist Health South Florida.

Thank you to Fareed Al-Mashat and Alla Katsenovich for their invaluable photography and design expertise. Fareed and Alla spent endless hours with Andra and me during the photography sessions, and at times we disagreed on how to best express a nursing attribute in a still photograph. I learned that Fareed's instincts are impeccable, and he was always correct. Fareed is a talented photographer, and I was very fortunate to have the opportunity to work with him.

I want to thank our chief nursing officers, who hosted *The Art of Nursing* photo exhibitions at their hospitals and presented these images to our employees. Thank you to our hospital CEOs for their support of this project.

Deborah Mulvihill encouraged me to undertake the photo exhibition as well as this book, and trusted me to see them through. Andra Ogden Demorizi coordinated the involvement of dozens of busy healthcare professionals across multiple locations, and her attention to detail kept the project moving forward. Georgina Gonzalez-Robiou lent her marketing and communications expertise to ensure a professional finished product. Sincere thanks to all of you.

Our graphic designer, Rhondda Edmiston, and editor, Timothy Dodson, deserve recognition for their role in giving an elegant form and structure to our book. We have worked closely together for so many months I feel almost as if they are part of the Baptist Health family.

I am grateful to the staff throughout Baptist Health who helped us capture these images — in particular, our nurse managers, who went out of their way to ensure that the nurses represented in these images were given the time to spend with us, as well as making available the work areas where the photographs were taken. I would like to recognize Suzanne Balbosa-Sauders, Baptist Hospital Emergency Care Department; Nancy Martinez, Homestead Hospital; Melanie O'Neill, Mariners Hospital; Deborah Thomas, Baptist Hospital, 4 Clarke; Magalie La Combe, South Miami Hospital, 3 East Tower; Simone Cheong, South Miami Hospital, 5 East Tower; Barbara Ames and Sally Bonet, South Miami Hospital Clinical Learning; Norma Sabates, Doctors Hospital Surgery; Jennifer Taylor, West Kendall Baptist Hospital Surgery; Bernie Arcena, West Kendall Baptist Hospital ICU; and the Reverend Michael Daily, Director of Community Ministries, Miami Baptist Association.

Finally, special thanks go to all the nurses whose images are immortalized on these pages. You gave freely of your time to come before the camera for hours. Likewise, thanks to those who took time to participate in interviews and share your thoughts about our profession. Your words are a wonderful complement to the images.

Yvonne Brookes, R.N.

ACKNOWLEDGMENTS

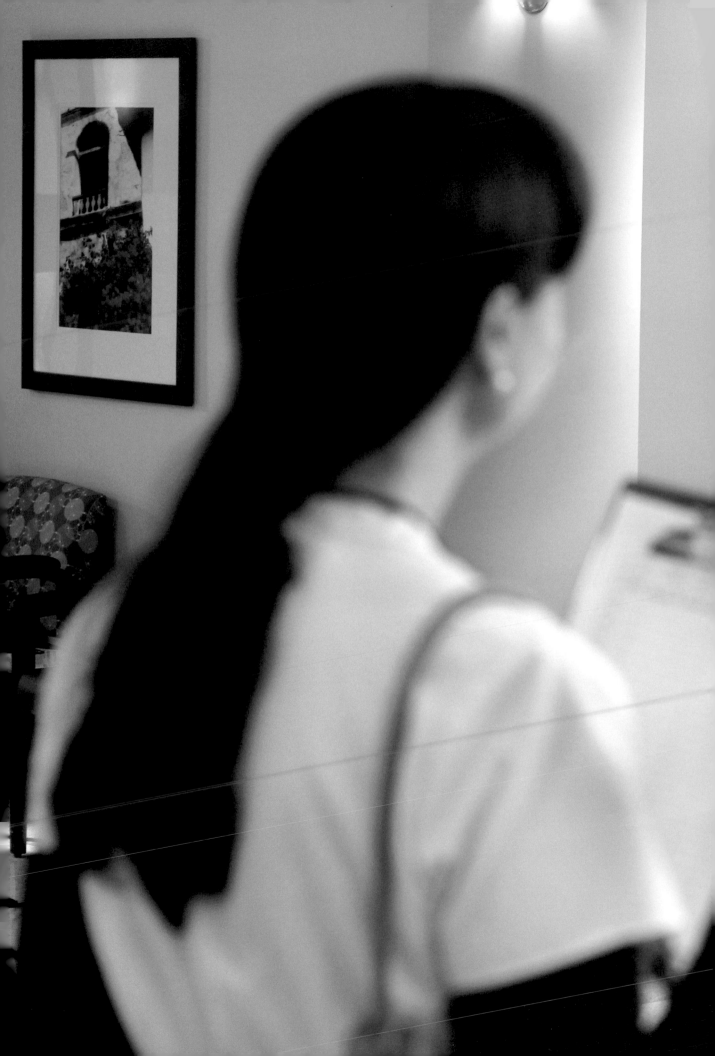

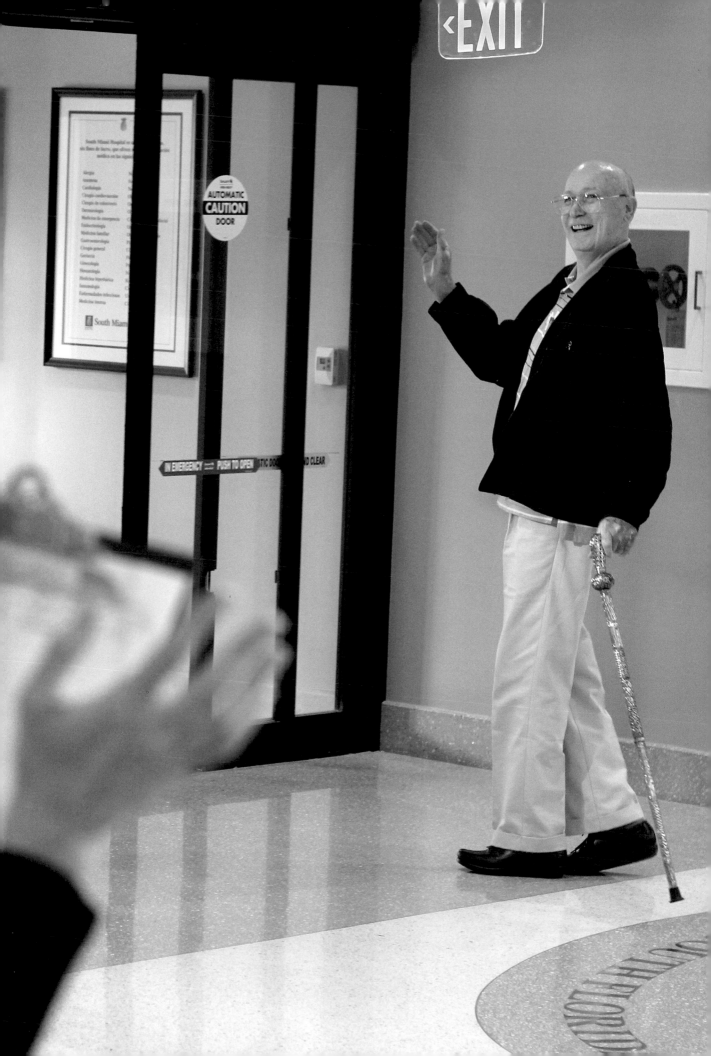

*The nurse, in all
professional relationships, practices
with compassion and respect
for the inherent dignity, worth,
and uniqueness of every individual,
unrestricted by considerations
of social or economic status,
personal attributes, or the nature
of health problems.*

*The nurse's primary commitment
is to the patient, whether
an individual, family, group,
or community.*

EXCERPT FROM THE "NURSING CODE OF ETHICS"